The Practice of Medicine

From Antiquity to Artificial Intelligence

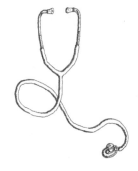

by
George Varghese, M.D.

Kansas City 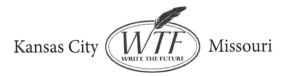 Missouri

The Practice of Medicine

From Antiquity to Artificial Intelligence

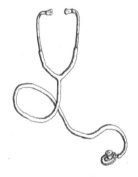

by
George Varghese, M.D.

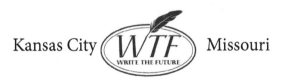

Kansas City **WTF** Missouri

WRITE THE FUTURE

Write the Future
Kansas City, Missouri

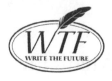

Copyright (C) 2021
George Varghese, M.D
First Edition 1 3 5 7 9 10 8 6 4 2
ISBN: 978-1-952411-59-5
LCCN: 2021933636

Editing: Martha McCarty
Design & Layout: w.e. leathem
Author contact: geovarghese@everestkc.net

Write the Future is an imprint of SPARTAN PRESS

Also by George Varghese, M.D.
To the Land of Opportunity: A Grandfather's Journey

Dedicated To

Molly. My loving wife of fifty years, mother of our three children and our source of support, encouragement and wise advice.

In Remembrance Of

My mother Anna. Teacher of a value system based on faith, morals, hard work and respect for others.

My grandmother Plamena. A believer in my potential throughout my life and hers.

Special Thanks

Dr. Sam Montello and Paul Stevens, tennis buddies, who buoyed my interest in writing medical history.

Dawn McInnis, Rare Book Librarian, who guided me in selection of books and assigned a room for intense research at Kansas University Medical Center's Clendening History of Medicine Library.

We strive for accuracy and fairness.
~ History Journal (online)

Facts and dates of ancient medical history are changeable, depending on the source and most current research. The intent is to be accurate.
~ George Varghese, M.D.

Contents

Twenty-First Century – *Computerized technology dominates*

The Future of Medicine

2020

MODERN MEDICINE
Does Medical History Matter?

Chapter One

Antiquity to Artificial Intelligence

Visit a doctor these days and chances are the physician will look at a computer screen and type notes while talking to you. There will be a cursory hands-on examination following this. The physician will then order an array of tests, arrive at a diagnosis and recommend a treatment plan.

This is not the way medicine had been practiced for thousands and thousands of years. Instead, it represents the metamorphosis of modern medicine from bedside to desktop. Is desktop medicine a threat to the ancient art of healing? As Google and Amazon push to manage health-care data, is the use of Artificial Intelligence/AI next on the horizon? Will a computerized system that mimics human intelligence, from visual perception to decision making and language translation assist us or replace us?

A growing reliance on technology is discussed in a subsequent chapter; first, let's review the where, when and how modern medicine evolved from simple to complex treatments, procedures, pioneering physicians and discoveries that stretch across the centuries, beginning as early as the third millennium B.C.

Imagine a region in an ancient world and a civilization considered to be advanced based on the tools they invented, homes and buildings they constructed and an irrigation system they developed to water crops. They created a written language and are thus considered to be a literate culture. Yet, one account of their history claimed there were no physicians. What then was the method of health care? What was the length of their lives? Did the civilization die out because there were no doctors? Or was the long-accepted record of a lack of medical history a misconception?

Consider also continents and cultures of early ages when medical practices were founded on religious beliefs and mythology. A prevailing belief was that diseases were sent by the gods as a form of punishment for sins. Globally, with the advance of civilizations through the ages, treatments and practices rooted in religion and mythology prevailed across the continents and countries and cities within. Much was governed by rulers, emperors, kings and priest-physicians, gods and demi-gods who devised methods of health care, relying on treatments (some which are used today), such as herbs, hymns, prayers, deep sleep like a form of hypnotism and interpretation of dreams.

As time marched on beyond B.C. to A.D., change came. New discoveries emerged in continents and civilizations within Asia to Europe and ultimately the Americas, North and South. Scientific research was conducted, textbooks were written, physicians taught what they had learned. The question is, does medicine of the past matter to us as modern practitioners? What lessons are buried in time gone by? For one, ancient medical discoveries still exist and are useful, thousands and thousands of years later. For another, Hippocrates' mantra Primum non nocer written in the 5th-century B.C. guides what we do today. Tools of the past—the stethoscope invented two-hundred years ago, for example, and the discovery of diabetes, percussion, papation and more laid a foundation for the practice of medicine in the 21st-century.

The unifying bond is this: Doctors have been entrusted with patient care and the quest to understand illness and heal patients throughout recorded history.

We are heirs of our predecessors' mission.

I have wondered, since I was a young student in India, who went before us? What were the influences and outcomes? As a physician, the history behind the vast range of medical discoveries from antiquity to Artificial Intelligence is of particular interest to me.

Not all the past history is written here. Sections are compiled to acknowledge an ever-changing advancement from medicine's once-slow, now accelerated, pace—from antiquity to the age of Artificial Intelligence.

5,000 - 500, B.C.

THE CRADLE OF CIVILIZATION
Civilization Begins

Chapter Two

Civilization Begins

At the end of the Ice Age 10,000 or so years ago and the beginning of the Neolithic Age (10,000-4500 B.C.), land turned fertile and green. Homo Sapiens who were hunter-gatherers until then became agriculturists and a new age of organized civilizations emerged. Among the earliest is Mesopotamia (5000-500 B.C.) known as the Cradle of Civilization based on its achievements. Inhabited by Sumerians, an Afro-Asiatic race, Mesopotamia advanced its civilization by building homes, temples, roads and wheeled methods of transportation, including chariots. They were first to document their history with characters carved on clay tablets, the ancient method of cuneiform. In that way, Sumerians created a written language and are acknowledged as having been literate.

With agriculture as a key to their survival, they raised livestock, such as pigs, goats and sheep, and grew wheat, barley and a variety of vegetables, including garlic and onions. Settled on land between the Euphrates and Tigris rivers (present day Iraq), Sumerians were inventive enough to devise an irrigation system to protect their crops from drought and feed their people.

Even today, as this book is written in the 21st-century, the artifacts of Mesopotamia continue to draw attention. An example is an exhibition, Mesopotamia: Civilization Begins, co-curated by Dr. Timothy Potts, director of the J. Paul Getty Museum in Los Angeles. The museum exhibit is divided into sections. Among them: First Cities. First Writings. First Kings.

But—was there no medical science and no art of healing? No physicians? No evidence of systematic health care in an advanced civilization?

The news that Mesopotamia existed without a health-care system was spread by Greek historian Herodotus (484-424 B.C.). Considered to be the Father of History as well as a philosopher and skilled physician, Herodotus wrote what he witnessed while traveling through Mesopotamia. He authored a series of books and, as reported in Medicine and Doctoring in Ancient Mesopotamia, Herodotus proclaimed: "They bring out all their sick into the streets, for they have no regular doctors. People that come along offer the sick man advice, either from what they personally have found to cure such a complaint, or what they have known someone else to be cured by. No one is allowed to pass by a sick person without asking what ails him."

However, "Herodotus's description of medical practice is categorically untrue," historian Emily K. Teall reported in the Grand Valley Educational Journal of History (2014). Based on Mesopotamia's own texts which were eventually translated and interpreted, the afflicted did not merely gather in the marketplace in hopes of a cure. Teall said: "Ill people may have very well discussed their ailments with neighbors on the street, but doctoring and places of recovery were far from non-existent, even including healing temples. Herodotus had the mindset of a medical tourist…and was likely more interested in exalting his own Greek culture than in taking an emic point of view."

Still, there is evidence that the Sumerian lifespan was not long. In the anthology Florilegium, 20th-century historian Leonard Churchin compiled reports on the life expectancy of the Sumerian race. According to Churchin's data, anthropologists examined seventeen skeletons and found only a few indicated the advanced age of sixty years. Average age was thirty-six years for males and twenty-eight for females. The reason for Sumerian's short lifespan may be unknown, but research has contradicted Herodotus' assumptions and eventually revealed new truths. Earlier, long before Churchin's and Teall's reports, a pair of researchers shed light on medical care in Mesopotamia by deciphering the clay tablets, the ancient cuneiform engravings.

An 18th-century German explorer, cartographer and scholar Carsten Niebuhr (1733-1815) decoded copies of cuneiform inscriptions discovered at Persepolis, today a World Heritage Site in Iran. Niebuhr is credited with "cracking the cuneiform code," leading to an understanding of the Sumerian people. He learned that doctors and practitioners in Mesopotamia were trained, had facilities and tools to treat patients with both pharmaceutical medicine and surgery, all integral to the advancement of the culture, according to Teall. Physician's equipment included surgical instruments and, though there were no large facilities that could be termed hospitals, the indication is that medical doctors treated patients, cared for the afflicted and belonged to an established profession. "Besides having offices, beds for patients, pharmacology and surgical equipment," Teall said, "Mesopotamian doctors had a professional name. Asu (or azu) were those who practiced therapeutic medicine, composed of surgical and herbal treatments."

Despite their skill and knowledge, a god of healing was supreme. Gula, a deity of healing and health was known as the "great physician of the black-headed ones," the Sumerians. Also associated with agriculture that is essential to survival, Gula was a patroness of doctors, healing arts and medical practices.

Further, in the 19th-century, Mesopotamia's cuneiform inscriptions were translated to English by Sir Henry Rawlinson (1810-1895), a Baronet of British descent. Proficient in the language spoken by Sumerians, Sir Rawlinson converted the inscriptions to a more-universal language. He earned the title Father of Assyriology, the historical and linguistic study of ancient cultures, and as reported in SciHi. org, a journal of science and art, trustees of the British Museum published four volumes of his cuneiform translations before his death.

Based on these revelations, what is it we can learn? That history is not always clear? What was once considered truth may be untrue in the future? What was believed to be the Gospel Truth may eventually be belittled and proven wrong? The uncertainty presents itself in medicine that is rooted in mythology of the future centuries.

Dates Uncertain

PRE-HISTORIC MEDICINE
Healers: The physicians or the gods?

Chapter Three

Medicine, Myths, Migration

A world map, had there been one, would have charted new continents, countries and cities built on land near rivers and seas in pre-historic times. Egypt, India, China and Greece formed cultures not known to have existed before. The new civilizations thrived and prospered and physicians administered health care for citizens and rulers. Still, their new world was not without the gods.

It is difficult to determine exact periods since ancient history was told orally through myths and legends, storytelling. With no written history and few actual dates, there was little proof until translation of Mesopotamia's cuneiform tablets and Egyptian hieroglyphics offered a glimpse of common methodologies. That is, skilled doctors treated the afflicted who gathered in temples, but they were not alone. Their counterparts, priest-physicians governed by gods directed treatments.

As it had been in Mesopotamia and continued to be in developing regions, health care and cures were administered by mortal doctors as well as gods of healing.

An unexplained commonality backed by scholars today is that pharaohs, kings, emperors and rulers, as well as physicians in ancient cultures, placed medical care in the hands of the gods. The ancient cultures shared a belief: Diseases were caused by demons.

Translation of Sumerian cuneiforms made of clay and Egyptian papyri written on material made from the papyrus plant categorized demons of various ailments, such as liver diseases, women's diseases, wasting and so on. Customarily, priest-physicians identified the particular demon and applied an appropriate remedy. Herbal medications were often prescribed, including irritants like garlic and asafetida drawn from the stem of fennel. Cascara, a strong laxative made from the bark of a tree, induced diarrhea intended to disgust the demon and ward it off the patient. Also common among the gods, according to the National Library of Medicine, was the belief that humans are a physical body of the earth and an invisible body of heaven. Whatever the illness, by the power of the gods (physicians, too), the diagnosis was that the disease was caused by a sin the patient had committed.

Illness, then, equaled sin. Doctoring, then, was tied to the mythological, supernatural and divine. The cure depended on the will of the gods.

The reason similarities and widespread commonalities in medical care flourished for centuries in dynasties and empires, from Egypt to India and Europe and the borders of China, can only be guessed or surmised.

How did it happen? Migration is a key.

With few exceptions, historians and scholars today theorize that seeds of organized human civilization were sown by Sumerians of Mesopotamia in the third millennium, then spread in all directions. Means of transport were developed, making it possible for populations to migrate beyond Mesopotamia, traveling through uncharted regions and infiltrating new continents and nations. Physicians, historians, scholars, students, traders and merchants rode on horses or in wheeled wagons and chariots drawn by oxen or donkeys for their expansive travel across continents. Though each new independent culture developed codes, laws, a social order and a separate language, Dr. John McWhorter, a renowned modern-day linguist, concludes that incoming populations learned the spoken language and were absorbed into the culture. In that way, they shared their history, their spiritual beliefs and their knowledge of medicine.

Most likely to justify the influence of a migration pattern is the Steppe Aryan culture developed in the Caucasus Mountain Valley between Caspian Sea and Black sea—Steppe denoting travel through dry, treeless terrain. Aryan speaking Proto-Indo-European language. As they migrated out of their homeland, the innovative Steppe Aryans took their concepts with them to Egypt, India, Greece and the borders of China. They spread their religion, philosophy, ideas and concepts of medicine, like those born in Mesopotamia.

Over a period of 1000 years or more, the Aryans branched out, traveling south, east and west, eventually migrating to other developed civilizations. Those who traveled southward found their way into northern India between 1500-500 B.C., the Vedic period. A 2018 edition of Early Indians: The Story of Our Ancestors by Tony Joseph highlights "threshold events" in which humans evolved to influence and alter complex societies. Joseph's history supports the premise (a theory I share) that defining events, such as the migration of Steppe Aryans tie history together. Cultural differences in ancient civilizations were established and yet, there were common methodologies in medicine, namely herbal pharmaceuticals and the practice hymns, prayers, incantations, amulets, deep sleep and interpretation of dreams.

Steppe Aryans had adapted an alphabet modeling Mesopotamia's Sumerian script and thus began one version of Sanskrit literature. Evidence supports that belief, but are the Steppe Aryans responsible for the common threads that ran through ancient medical practices? There are indications that commonality of medical practice in civilizations existed. I suspect—without written documentation, I can only suspect—the Steppe migration contributed to medical practice throughout ancient civilizations. The new nations were so far apart geographically, how could they have had the same philosophies and practices about medicine, including primitive methods of surgery? After extensive research and based on common methodologies within new civilizations, my own assumption is the migrants were the influence that connected them. If so, as history implies, the Steppe Aryan migration was a major threshold event in the history of medicine.

Ancient methods of healing would eventually give way to educated physicians, research and scientific discoveries. But not until after the phenomena of widespread commonalities in medical care flourished for centuries in dynasties and empires governed by rulers, pharaohs, emperors and kings. And the gods.

Read on about medicine in new civilizations. Begin with Egypt's contributions to modern medicine and the tragedy of King Tut, his deadly ailments, his physician and Sekhmet, a vengeful goddess of plagues and healing.

B.C. and Beyond

ANCIENT MEDICINE WORLDWIDE
Medicine of the new civilizations

Chapter Four

Medicine After Mesopotamia

Egypt

Much in the practice of medicine in the pre-historic period was unique, different between one civilization to another. Much was the same. And much is a reflection of modern medicine today. Such is true of Egypt.

For thousands of years, a continuing thread traced to Mesopotamia ran through medicine in ancient cultures. In each advanced civilization, a delicate balance of power existed between physicians, the gods of healing and the rulers, emperors, queens and kings.

Realistically, Egypt is modernized, leaving ancient remains to tourists, scholars and historians, though several of their medical discoveries are vital today because, says Valentina Bonev at California's Loma Linda Medical Center, "many ancient methods aren't so ancient after all. They are tried and true."

Tied to Egyptian medicine and still significant in modern medicine is transsphenoidal surgery. The minimally-invasive procedure is used today to access the brain through the nose to remove tumors. According to Raj Sindwani, an otolaryngologist at Ohio's Cleveland Clinic, ancient Egyptians discovered the easiest access point to the brain was through the nose and the sphenoid sinus. Ebers papyrus, a translation of Egyptian written texts, depict the Egyptian process of inserting a long, hooked implement through the nostril to break the thin bone of brain case and remove the brain through the nose. Why? To disarm the brain as an unimportant organ in the embalming (mummification) process. But the heart, believed to be the center of emotion, thought and soul was preserved to be useful in the afterlife.

A lesser example of an ancient influence in modern medicine is leeching. In Egyptian medicine, leeches—worms with suckers at both ends—sucked blood through the skin and, unappealing as it seems, medicinal leeches are in demand in medicine today. The U.K. Telegraph headlined leeching as a "wacky new celebrity anti-aging treatment." But America's Food and Drug Administration/FDA has approved medicinal leeches for reconstructive and plastic surgery. Doctors today are known to prescribe leeches for a host of ailments, including varicose veins and blocked arteries and badly infected areas. According to a current report by the Science History Institute, "Leech saliva contains a chemical called hirudin, a natural anticoagulant."

The Cesarean Section/C-section, a medical procedure that is commonplace today is also referenced in ancient history. Success of the Cesarean Section in ancient Egypt is undocumented, but according to America's Centers for Disease Control and Prevention, nearly one-third of all babies born in the U.S. today are delivered by C-Section and globally, the numbers are rising. Reported by CNN:Health, the highest number of C-Sections are performed in America, Italy, Switzerland and Germany with the fewest performed in India and Africa.

Physicians of Egypt, with few exceptions, were males who were practiced in setting bones and dislocated joints, but performed no surgery except for circumcision, common at the time to mark the passage from childhood to adulthood. Ebers papyrus also detailed Egyptian characteristics, cases and treatment for mental disorders, such as dementia and depression. However, mental illness was viewed as an influence of evil spirits and angry gods.

Some scholars rank Egyptian medicine as surprisingly sophisticated, yet doctors and rulers who wore the crown interacted with the gods and appeased them through religious rituals and offerings. The sick gathered in healing temples and were treated with prayers, incantations and cures sent by deities. Doctors considered to be priest-physicians were chosen by the king. Religious clergy and the kings were then go-betweens the people and the healing gods. Among them was a powerful and vengeful deity Sekhmet, a mythological goddess of plagues and healing. Her dual nature brought disease to those who wronged her and also, at her will, granted cures to ailments she had delivered.

While medical history was made in Egypt, not all methodologies ended well. Papyrus recorded repugnant and deadly treatments, including animal dung ointments and dead mouse paste. A CBS television presentation on the history of ancient medicine asked: "Who'd put a dead mouse in their mouth? The Egyptians did. In doing so, the hope was to ease toothache. In some cases, mashed mouse was blended with other ingredients and the resulting poultice was applied to the painful spot." A Sumerian practice of bloodletting—

evidence that Steppe Aryan migration influenced medicine beyond Mesopotamia—was a common procedure which often resulted in accidental death from blood loss.

Every-day life elixirs in Egypt were made of honey oil, castor oil and herbal concoctions. Copper was used to sterilize wounds and drinking water. Recognizing the importance of pulse in diagnoses, Egyptians are said to have measured it by count and characteristics, regular or irregular, strong or weak. They may have introduced palpation (feeling with hands). The word palpation was not used, but records show touching was part of an examination. Tomb paintings in Egypt depict individuals being massaged or "kneaded" like bread dough.

None, neither the gods nor the priests and physicians, could save Egypt's eternally-famous Tutankhamon, King Tut, the Golden Boy King (1305-1324 B.C.). When his tomb was pried open in 1922 after being sealed for 3200 years, modern forensics revealed King Tut suffered from malaria, fractured bones and congenital deformities associated with inbreeding. He rose to the throne at age nine and died at age nineteen.

Written documentation decoded and translated to interpret Egyptian history includes the Edwin Smith papyrus (1700 B.C.) named for the American Egyptologist and translated to English in 1920 by university professor James Henry Breasted, also an American Egyptologist. Ebers Papyrus (1550 B.C.) is named for German Egyptologist George Ebers who purchased the original scroll in 1873. Rosetta Stone (196 B.C.) is a 1799 discovery found in the Nile Delta. French scholar Jean-Francois Champollion (1790-1832) is credited with deciphering the hieroglyphics in 1822.

Not all medical mysteries were buried in cuneiform tablets and papyrus scrolls. As noted in the next chapter, India's medical history recorded in Vedic Sanskrit is viewed as a modern-day revelation.

Chapter Five

Knowledge of Life

India

The theory of Steppe Aryans influencing the practice of medicine in ancient civilizations as long as 3000 years ago may be best illustrated in India. Four Vedas written in Sanskrit are believed to have been told orally by early Aryans who migrated to India. One of four Vedas is dedicated to medicine. It reveals that common treatments for healing and preservation of health were prayers to various gods and herbal medications, diet and exercises, perhaps yoga. Atharva Veda further describes diseases like tumors, abscesses, heart disease, diarrhea and constipation. These writings formed the basis for Ayurveda (knowledge of life).

Ayurvedic medicine is reported to be the oldest medical system in the world. However ancient, it is not obsolete. In India, Ayurveda is accepted as a form of medical care, equal to conventional Western medicine, traditional Chinese medicine and homeopathic medicine, according to a Johns Hopkins Medical Report. Practitioners in India undergo state-recognized, institutional training. Ayurvedic medicine is also practiced in institutions throughout Europe, America and Latin America.

However ancient, Ayurvedic medicine is not obsolete, but there is history behind it. The highest development of ancient medicine in India occurred during the Brahman period (800 B.C. - 100 A.D.), named for the Hindu god, Brahma. Three of the greatest physicians of that era were Sushruta, Charaka and Vagbhata. Before them was Atreya, the chosen physician to King Nagnajita of the ancient Gandhara Kingdom. Atreya attended the king. In the city of Taxila, Atreya taught medicine at Taxila University, one of the oldest universities in world history.

Sushruta and Charaka were disciples of Atreya whose Atreya Samhita, a compendium of disease, divided diseases as those that can be cured and those that cannot be cured. Sushruta Samhita, a surgical document, identified eleven-hundred diseases and seven-hundred herbal medicines. Sushruta Samhita described several surgical procedures and instruments, such as scissors, forceps, needles and sutures.

Charaka Samhita was a medical treatise. Charaka discussed three humors (life forces) called Vata (mental and physical); Pitta (metabolic) and Kapha (lubrication of bodily parts and systems). When in balance there was health. When one was deficient or in excess, there was disease. Treatment focused on ways to regain and maintain balance. Charaka also described five-hundred different herbal plants used as medication.

Spices and herbs were plentiful while I was growing up in India. Turmeric, a popular herb used in modern cultures today, my family used as a spice. We didn't know the medical value at the time. Now there is scientific evidence to support its effectiveness in treating inflammation, joint pain and infections. Healthline advises that to feel the full anti-inflammatory effect, choose a supplement that contains significant amounts of curcumin, the main active ingredient in turmeric.

The third noted Indian physician of the period was Vagbhata, a follower of Charaka. His treatise Astanga Samgraha discussed therapeutics. According to Vagbhata, nature can take care of many ailments and eighty-five percent of diseases can be cured without a doctor. Only fifteen percent require a doctor. A sayings in modern medicine reflects Vagbhata's premise. That is to watch. To be sure there are no complications. To let nature take its course.

Still, the gods were not to be ignored in Indian medicine. Lord Indra, god in Vedic mythology, was a powerful overseer of the healing gods. Legends claim that Indra gave knowledge to Dhanvantari, Hindu physician god of healing. Hinduism Today reports that countless numbers, millions, still visit a sacred 5000-year-old temple in Kerala in search of blessings and cures. The faithful form a pilgrimage, walking from all over southern India and going up and up and up to a temple on a hill.

Though ancient, Indian methodologies, such as Yoga and massage have been passed down over thousands of years and are widely-used now. The British Broadcasting Company/BBC noted that Charaka believed impurities absorbed from the surrounding environment should be cleansed through sweating. He advised perspiring by way of steaming to purify yourself. Today? The steam room or the sauna at a spa would be the place to go.

Ayurvedic medicine, a natural and holistic approach to physical and mental health, has been adopted world-wide with the exception of America. For the past two decades, as cited in the U.S. National Library of Medicine, the Foundacion Salud dy Ayurved Prema Argentina offers courses in the School of Medicine of the University of Buenos Aires and the National University of Cordoba's School of Medicine. The same is true in several European countries. In America, Ayurvedic institutions are viewed with skepticism. The Johns Hopkins report points out that Ayurvedic practitioners are generally not licensed in the United States, nor is there a national standard for Ayurvedic training or certification. In 2007, America's Food and Drug Administration/FDA banned certain Ayurvedic products, warning that one in five Ayurvedic medicines contain toxic metals, like lead, mercury and arsenic. The Johns Hopkins conclusion: Ayurveda can have positive effects when used as a complementary therapy in combination with standard, conventional medical care. In other words, consult your physician.

Without question, medical treatments through the ages have been brilliant or sometimes bizarre. Notable discoveries, beliefs and practices have been embraced or, just as frequently, spurned. This question lingers: Does history of medicine matter? The answer is yes. Though historically archaic, buried wisdom handed down from the ancients has a niche in a modern age. Throughout history, medical practice is tied to the common goal of healing, as evidenced in Egypt, India and in the following chapter, China.

Chapter Six

Ancient but Modern?

China

New scientific advancements and innovative techniques were unknown in ancient civilizations, such as China, yet some medical mainstays have been carried over from China to modern medicine worldwide. Thousands and thousands of years have passed since China developed its methodologies, including the ancient theory of Yin and Yang—the interdependence between two opposing forces—but has the concept survived time? And has the belief that snake oil is "a cure for what ails you" regained authenticity today? Perhaps... or perhaps not.

Let's begin at the beginning. The Classic Canon of Medicine was written during China's Chen dynasty (likely 557-589 A.D.) and the Canon named the heart as Prince of the Body and the Seat of Vital Spirit. Lungs were the origin of breath and liver, the dwelling place of soul. As aids to diagnoses, History-taking and observation of a patient's abnormal signs mirror practices of Egypt and India as do using palpation of affected areas and placing importance on pulse rate, strength and regularity.

As in other ancient cultures, Chinese medicine was also anchored to the belief that diseases were caused by demons of the body and demons of the mind.

Healing was performed in temples by priest-physicians and treatments included incantations, words chanted as a magic spell, and amulets, ornaments believed to be protection against evil spirits and disease.

In Chinese mythology, Shennong (between 300-201 B.C.) is a deity thought to be Father of Traditional Chinese Medicine. He was worshipped as a patron god and as one of Three Kings, legendary emperor deities. Shennong created a detailed catalog listing three-hundred-sixty-five botanical medicines and he was known to try his own herbal medicines. A report in Mytholopedia said Shennong met his untimely death after ingesting a poisonous plant in one of his own concoctions.

Equally respected was Lao Tzu (age unknown) who believed in Yin and Yang, cosmic forces in the body. Harmony between the two forces assured health and lack of it caused illness. Acupuncture, massage and herbal medicines were presented as ways to regain balance; hygiene was an important element of treatment, too. There were greater and lesser natural elements, like wood, fire, earth, metal and water which controlled the cosmic forces. Corresponding to each element was an organ, including liver, heart, lungs and kidneys.

First discovered in Egypt and China, massage (sports massage included) is a mainstream therapy practiced internationally in the 21st-century. Acupuncture developed in China approximately 4000 years ago, has spread as an alternative treatment worldwide. Modern-day acupuncture enthusiasts profess that carefully placed acupuncture needles help balance Yin and Yang. During the past forty years, acupuncture and massage, the therapeutic techniques of oriental medicine, have surged in popularity. Massage is commonplace and according to the U.S National Library of Medicine, more than ten million acupuncture treatments are administered annually in the United States alone. Acupuncture's rise in popularity is linked to its effectiveness for pain relief and to the fact that scientific studies have begun to prove its benefits, the library reported.

Numerous references to Cesarean Section appear in ancient China's history, the U.S. National Library of Medicine has reported. Chinese etchings depict the procedure on apparently living women. Yet, the National Library pointed out, early history of Cesarean Section in Egypt and China remain shrouded in myth and is of dubious accuracy. So it was that the ancient Chinese believed in an abundance of methodologies, but the supernatural, such as clairvoyance and the power of gods were common beliefs, too. In most cultures today, the status of mythological gods to govern medicine has rescinded. But what of Chinese snake oil and the "cosmic force" of Yin and Yang?

In the 19th- and 20th-century, traveling Snake Oil Salesmen were characterized as quacks or charlatans in American "cowboy movies" and in Mark Twain's Huckleberry Finn. But a recent Scientific American report carried the headline: Snake Oil Salesman Were Onto Something! Whether it be for arthritis, heart disease or possibly depression, snake oil is a cure, the report by Cynthia Graber claimed. Could it be?

Known as a remedy in Chinese medicine

to treat joint pain, such as arthritis and bursitis, its introduction to the U.S. is traced to Chinese laborers who built the Transcontinental Railroad and suffered aches and pains of hard physical labor in the 1800s. Meanwhile, nutritional research by California's Richard Kunin (1935 -) concluded that snake oil has been part of Western medicine since the time of the Sumerians 4000 years ago. Published in the Western Journal of Medicine, Dr. Kunin reported that Chinese water-snake oil contains a higher percent of Omega-3 fatty acids than the popular food source, salmon. Snake oil is sold over-the-counter internationally. But prescribed by physicians? Unlikely.

Practitioners backed by studies of acupuncture say yes, acupuncture is therapeutic and widely used today. Meanwhile, Yin and Yang, a concept embedded in ancient Chinese medicine is often heard in modern-day vernacular, but dismissed in a Science Forum report. Yin and Yang, the report concluded, is not a viable scientific theory. It is merely a way of looking at things.

History of medicine constantly evolves and is often questioned, as evidenced by Greek physicians Hippocrates and Galen.

Chapter Seven

Science and the Supernatural

Greece

Alexander the Great (356-323 B.C.), King of the Greek Kingdom of Macedon, was a student of Aristotle (385-323 B.C.) and adopted aspects of Aristotle's science and theories of Greek medicine. Similar to, yet in some ways different than the Egyptians, Indians and Chinese, Greeks considered the human heart to be the most important organ of the body, the seat of intelligence, emotion and sensation.

Alexander accepted Aristotle's findings as valid and recognized the significance of skilled physicians. Though he was knowledgeable about medicine, he was known to have worshipped a mythical god. So it happened that Greek medicine mixed religion, science and mythology to serve the people and the king. Alexander chose Philippos of Acarnania (age uncertain) as his personal physician and legend has it that Alexander trusted the skill, honesty and friendship of Philippos. Still, he placed faith in Asclepius, god of healing, and sanctified two-hundred healing temples (Asclepeions) dedicated to Asclepius.

Priest-physicians in Grecian temples relied on religion, superstition and supernatural methods for healing. As in other powerful civilizations, herbal elixirs were used along with incantations and amulets, as if they were magic. Greek mythology sanctified Hypos, the Greek god of sleep who induced a form of hypnosis and interpreted dreams to aid a diagnosis.

In images and paintings, the god Asclepius holds a staff with a serpent entwined around it, the symbol of medicine even today. Though he was revered in Homer's Iliad and other writings, Asclepius is a lesser god, a demi-god, son of Apollo and Coronis, a mortal (scandalous) woman.

Theoretically, both physical and psychological health were prized by Greek Macedonians and some health problems were rooted in the belief that illness was caused by "bad blood." As did many physicians of ancient medicine, Greek physicians practiced bloodletting, cutting open a vein to let bad blood drain. While bloodletting likely began with Sumerians and Egyptians, it became a common practice in Greek medicine. In many nations then and still today, leeches were also used to suck blood through the skin.

Two reports of the great Alexander and ancient Greek medicine have since been questioned or considered faulty. One, though unsubstantiated, is that Alexander died of alcoholic liver disease, fever and strychnine poisoning. Yet recently, a research scholar at the University of Maryland College of Medicine said it is more likely Alexander died of typhoid fever or malaria, deadly conditions at the time.

In regard to obstetrics, most ancient Greek writers speak highly of midwives and Greek philosopher Socrates himself proudly stated he was the son of a midwife, a much respected profession of the era, according to the Journal of Prenatal and Life Sciences. Additionally, the scholarly paper, Caesarian Section in Ancient Greek Mythology notes that Caesarian birth appears in Greek mythology on several occasions. Myth, though, is a spoken narrative transmitted from one generation or one culture to another, thus its veracity is unknown. Other reports claim that while influenced by Greek medicine, Caesarean Section is named for the Roman statesman Julius Caesar (60 B.C.). That, however, is a common misconception and completely without merit, says United Nations of Roman Victrix/UNRV.

Also disputed is that the Greek's understanding of the heart preceded Egyptians. Long ago, Scientific Corroborations of Theosophy, published in 1909, Dr. A. Marques was adamant, almost defiant, in his claim: Egyptian papyri make intelligent references to the heart, blood vessels, pulse and circulation of blood. The views of the ancient Greeks on circulation of blood were almost exactly those which the Egyptians had taught many centuries earlier. It was not Greece, therefore, but Egypt that was the "motherland of rational medicine and anatomy."

What remains without dispute is that through all of time, change occurs, yet the common bond of medicine is to heal. Beyond Mesopotamia, commonalities in the practice of medicine were evident in Egypt, India, China and Greece. Still today, gods are super powers in Africa, Tibet and other East Asian countries where ceremonial rituals and singing and dancing to appease evil spirits continues. After as many as 5000 years, fervent prayer to the Christian God or a god of choice is a plea for hope and healing. Around the world, families, friends and neighbors form prayer circles to pray for healing. In my forty years as a practitioner, I encouraged faith as part of the healing process in a bad situation, such as spinal injury.

Belief in the domain of mythological gods and deities endured in ancient cultures. But change will come.

Chapter Eight

Change Came

At a time when citizens, physicians and kings attributed sickness to superstition and the wrath of the gods, Greek physician Hippocrates (460-370 B.C.) did not.

Hippocrates challenged prevailing beliefs that diseases are caused by supernatural forces with cures governed by mythological gods. By way of Hippocrates, change came gradually, but certainly, to the practice of medicine in Greece and other lands.

Regarded as the Father of Medicine, Hippocrates remains today as one of the most, perhaps the most, influential figures in the history of medicine. He lived for ninety years, much of his life during the reign of Alexander the Great. Research shows he was a physician in the Greek healing temple Askolepian on the island of Cos. Yet during his lifetime, he espoused the theory that diseases are the result of natural causes, rather than deities, and treatment should be by natural methods.

He is credited with developing the theory of four humors, vital bodily fluids, identified as:

- Blood

- Phlegm

- Yellow bile

- Black bile

With careful History-taking and observation, it was then up to the physician to detect an excess or deficiency of any of these, correct it and re-establish balance between the humors for health and prevention of disease.

As many as sixty textbooks written by Hippocrates have survived the centuries, according to Encyclopedia Brittanica. Today, dozens of books compile Hippocrates' writings on signs, symptoms of diseases, diagnosis, treatment, prognosis and more. His books detailed History-taking and observation for abnormal signs. He took medical practice out of temples and taught ways to detect which humor was out of balance. He also linked health to the influence of earth, air, water, fire and qualities of dryness, cold and heat. Heredity, climate, body constitution and geography played a role in the incidence of sickness and disease. Hippocrates' Materia Medica detailed a number of herbal treatments made from gifts of nature, leaves, seeds and flowers.

The Father of Medicine's teachings spread world-wide and have defied time. Even in a modern world, the Hippocratic Oath written 2500 years ago is recited by students entering medical school. The oath is viewed as a promise to uphold the art of medicine and act in the patient's interest. David Katz, M.D. at Yale University has said, "Hippocrates was a visionary who figured out important ways to stay healthy, all of which have been proven by modern science and have helped shape modern medicine."

Though Hippocrates is acclaimed, even exalted, in the history of medicine, translations of ancient Sanskrit texts from India and medical texts from Egypt and China cast a shadow of doubt on his status of being first in methods of health and wellness. A prime example is that in India, Charaka medical students recited an oath similar to the Hippocratic oath when pupils were accepted for training. To say this is to raise a question: Do translations of ancient scripts suggest that Hippocrates could be accurately categorized as the Father of Western Medicine, but not medicine of the entire world?

Nevertheless, he lives in history as a paragon. His clinical contributions to medicine are viable today as is one of his most basic concepts. That is: Walking, a natural method of treatment, is the healthiest form of exercise. Theoretically, Hippocrates was among the first to note that those who are sedentary have far more health problems than those who are active. He also recognized that patients who become overweight are more likely to have serious health problems. He is cited as saying, "Everything in excess is opposed to nature." Today, it's "Everything in moderation."

By following the teachings of Hippocrates, another famous Greek physician from ancient times emerged as a great diagnostician and renown practitioner (noted in the next chapter). He is Claudius Galen.

Chapter Nine

A Science And An Art

The timeless premise that medicine is a science and an art is traced to Greek physician Claudius Galen (130-210 A.D.), the first known to espouse the concept. Among eminent physicians from ancient times—second only to his predecessor Hippocrates (460-370 B.C.)—Galen professed the art of healing was intended to use logos (reason and rational knowledge) in conjunction with experience. He established himself as a respected diagnostician and popularized the use of physical signs for diagnoses by professing, according to medical historians, that science provides the knowledge of what is healthy, unhealthy or intermediate; however, diagnoses are not based on intellectual knowledge and logos alone. His premise was founded on his belief that making a diagnosis involves perception by practice and experience with the additional powers of an educated guess (and intuition)—a form of art.

Few had greater influence on medical practice than Galen during his lifetime and on through the Middle Ages (500-1000 A.D.) Though of Greek descent, he forged his reputation in Rome, first as a physician treating Roman gladiators' combat wounds, thereby earning the attention of Roman Emperor Marcus Aurelius (121-180 A.D.). Galen was then summoned and appointed as the personal physician to the emperor who reigned during fifteen years of Rome's deadly Antonine Plague—also known as the Plague of Galen (as he supposedly named it at the outset).

In addition to being a master diagnostician, Galen was equally renown as a clinician, surgeon, philosopher, and an educator who taught abnormal physical signs of diseases. Earlier physicians—namely Greek physician Hippocrates and Indian doctors Sushruta and Charaka—discussed and theorized diseases, prognoses and treatments, yet scholarly journals credit Galen as being first to emphasize the importance of physical signs coupled with the art of healing in making a diagnosis.

In Galen's written works he, like Hippocrates, professed that nature has a bearing in curing illnesses and the cause of diseases were not tied to supernatural forces. Certain things nature can accomplish was his belief. In other situations, physicians aid nature. Recorded accounts describe his foundation for making diagnoses was to gather information by History-taking and apply the skills of observation, reasoning, exploration and the senses. Among Galen's procedures to help diagnosis and unite science and the art of healing are these:

General Observation: Posture, breathing pattern, color of skin, color of mucosa, color of eyes, urine, stool and other indicators, such as walking gait, pattern of movement and facial expressions.

Tactile Exploration: Touch to detect a mass for size, tenderness, swelling, temperature and regularity and volume of pulse rate. Galen introduced and promoted palpation—hands-on examination.

Sensory Observation: Hearing, seeing, touching, smelling and, though rarely, tasting.

Scholarly Reasoning: Scientific evidence, knowledge, experience and logic.

In limitations of the time, there was no way for Galen to assess the status of internal organs. Dissection of human cadavers was not allowed in ancient medicine. While dissection had once been practiced and then abandoned in ancient Greece, religious taboos inhibited ancient physicians, such as

Galen from "opening the human body for an-atomical purposes," according to literature in the U.S. National Library of Medicine.

Alternatively, in determination to un-derstand anatomy, Galen dissected animals and from that inferred what would be hu-man anatomy. He authored an estimated one-hundred-fifty textbooks during his life-time. Though many were lost, his texts and teachings on anatomy and physiology were followed as if they were the Gospel Truth and his influence, reported on ABC/UK, reigned supreme for fifteen centuries.

It was not until scientific research of two prominent physicians in the Renaissance Age questioned Galen's reign. Belgian anatomist Andreas Vesalius (1514-1564) dissected hu-man corpses and published an influential book on human anatomy that altered Galen's teachings. Similarly, English physician Wil-liam Harvey (1578-1657) refuted Galen's un-derstanding of circulation. Both Vesalius and Harvey met with resistance from academia before their research on anatomy and physi-ology was accepted because correcting Galen was unthinkable at the time.

That Galen's teachings on anatomy and physiology were eventually examined and de-termined to be incorrect is understandable.

His studies were based on dissection of pigs and monkeys, not human cadavers. Still, that discoveries he made informed the practice of medicine for hundreds and hundreds of years after his death is indisputable. And his assertion that the practice of medicine as a science and an art has endured for centuries. Only now in a digital age, is it questioned.

Over time, Galen's assumptions on circulation were eventually altered. He had taught that there are three interconnected systems in the body: brain and nerves, heart and arteries and liver and veins. He professed that liver produced venous blood which carried nutrients to various part of the body. Blood went from heart to lungs for oxygenation and then to the brain which was responsible for sensations. A fallacy was that blood did not return to heart and was consumed by the body. This prompted him to recommend bloodletting and enemas as a form of treatment. These teachings went uncontested for fifteen-hundred years, as did his understanding of human anatomy.

So devoted were his followers, that few discredited his findings. Even da Vinci whose anatomical drawings were superior, didn't say anything negative about Galen. For me, Galen is my hero, partly because he emphasized bedside examination, the art of healing. I admire him and hold him in esteem as many practitioners still do.

The influence of Hippocrates in Galenic medicine cannot be overlooked, but I am among those who say without Galen's contributions, medicine would not be what it is today. Yet, medical practice and discoveries are ever-changing as evidenced in the following era, the Middle Ages.

480-1300, A.D.

MEDICINE IN THE MIDDLE AGES
Scientists and physicians enlighten the Dark Ages

Chapter Ten

Medicine and the Monasteries

After the fall of the Roman Empire, historians and scholars commonly called the Middle
Ages (500-1500 A.D.) the Dark Ages. Often
dismissed as lacking knowledge and advancement, research now reveals significant devel-
opments, ranging from a collection of medical texts and, over time, hospitals, universities
and predominance of Christianity throughout Europe.

Most significant is the contribution
Benedictine monks made to medicine and
the culture. Founded by Benedict (480-543
A.D.), an Italian educated in Rome, compulsory reading elevated monastic monks'
literacy and monasteries became, said History World, "great centres of learning." Later,
by the Rule of Benedict (canonized as Saint
Benedict in 1964), copying texts, primarily
those of Greek physicians Hippocrates and

Galen, was added as another compulsory task. Writing on parchment made from the skin of sheep or goats, scribes used a quill, the shaft of a bird feather. Also innovative was the source of black ink drawn from a cocoon where wasps laid their eggs on oak trees.

By hand copying medical texts, monks, doctors and students relied on them to expand their knowledge. Near a Benedictine Abbey in Salerno, Italy, the monks established a hospital for the sick and by the year 1000, founded Salerno medical college, Schola Medica Salernitana. The first of its kind in the world, the full-fledged medical school devised a curriculum for both didactic and clinical training as well as graduation requirements for doctors of medicine. The Prized Writing Project at University of California, Davis, noted that monks practiced medicine, too. Monastic libraries built medical collections that served to train monk-practitioners about physiological systems of the arteries, veins, bones and muscles. Abbots, heads of monasteries—"men of great learning and great holiness"—often used their authority to appoint a monk as chief physician.

Before they copied medical texts, monks had copied biblical texts and spread the message of Christian religion. With that, medical traditions changed to written texts and allegiance, not to the gods of mythology, but to a powerful monolithic deity, the Christian God and Christian theology, prayer and the will of God as the basis of their beliefs.

The danger of bacteria and uncleanliness had not yet been realized and deadly diseases such as smallpox, cholera, syphilis and wound infections spread and were treated with medicinal plants and alkaloids like those of ancient Greece and India. As more medical schools were founded, education became formal and organized throughout Europe and the use of medical textbooks increased.

The controversy, if there was one, would be that monasteries, particularly of the Benedictine Order, tried and emphatically did, control medicine in the Middle Ages. With the benefit of their knowledge came the power to teach, care for the sick and govern the practice of medicine tied to their theology. Yet the belief that Christianity stunted the advancement of science in the Middle Ages is bogus, said James Hannam PhD, professor of History and Philosophy of Science at University of Cambridge, UK. In his book, God's Philosophers: How the Medieval World Laid the Foundation of Modern Science (2010), he claimed the Church insisted that science and mathematics were compulsory studies. "Of course," he wrote, "modern genetics was founded by a future Abbot growing peas in the monastic garden." The Austrian monk Gregor Mendel (1822-1884) is credited with the discovery and is titled Father of Modern Genetics. Mendel's discovery occurred soon after the Middle Ages, yet Dr. Hannam concluded, maybe the Dark Ages weren't so dark after all.

Simultaneously during the period, allopathic medicine advanced in Europe while ancient medicine maintained its prominence in other parts of the world. Ancient Chinese medicine endured and Ayurvedic medicine dating back to 2000 B.C. continued as the foundation of medical practice in India (my homeland). It is fortunate that the two-hundred-year dominance of British colonists (18th-20th-century) did not destroy the Indian form of medicine as it did India's industrial base and rich trade of silk, cotton, tea and spices.

In the time between the Late Middle Ages and the Renaissance, Germany's Gutenberg press fulfilled a greater demand for books. The press printed 3600 pages a day compared to forty pages a day, hand copied by monks. More and more pages of medical history were published and medical textbooks became widely available. With them came new ideas.

Chapter Eleven

It Is Written

Factual and unquestioned for centuries were the textbooks on anatomy, physiology, diseases, diagnoses and treatments written by Galen, a respected Greek physician of the 2nd-century. His writings served as primary teaching materials for 1500 years. Especially those on anatomy and physiology, Galen's texts were accepted as if they were Gospel Truth. However, other notable books were written by physicians during the Middle Ages and ultimately, Galen's work was questioned.

Reflecting on this brings a memory of an incident from my practice days at a leading academic hospital in the Midwest. I was asked to see a patient in the neurosurgical unit. A middle-aged man with uncontrollable muscle spasm from neck to legs had been admitted. The pattern was highly unusual. Scans and tests were negative. When I walked into the room with my intern, the patient was standing at the bedside, holding onto the grab bar. He was conscious and talking, but was arched backward like a bow. Watching him, my thought process flashed back to my medical school days and two catchy words I had learned and remembered: Opisthotonos and Risus Sardonicus—a characteristic description of tetanus diagnosed by an ancient writer!

When I walked out of the room, I told the intern, "If I were in India, I would say this man has tetanus." I couldn't imagine seeing a tetanus patient in a big city.

"Well, we are exhausted with all the tests," said the neurosurgeon who had heard me mention tetanus. "Why not order a tetanus titer?"

The test came back positive and the patient was successfully treated. (Usual treatment is vaccine, antibiotics and easing the muscle spasm.) The ancient author of the text I remembered was prominent Greek physician Aretaeus of Cappadocia (age uncertain; likely the 2nd-century). History places Aretaeus as one of the greatest medical scholars of antiquity. He wrote books on causes and symptoms of acute diseases, chronic diseases and therapeutics. He is known for vivid descriptions in his work. He wrote the earliest accounts of asthma, epilepsy, pneumonia, uterus cancer, diphtheria, tetanus and he gave diabetes its name, according to a report by the U.S. National Library of Medicine. He described diabetes as a disease that caused unquenchable thirst, excessive drinking and frequent urination, calling it diabetes from the Greek word siphon, water in water out. The memory reinforced my belief that much of what we learn from ancient medicine is relevant today.

Other memorable pioneering physicians from Greece, Italy, Britain, Switzerland and Persia (now Iran) also penned medical texts used to teach and educate doctors and students. Among the most notable of the early Christian era was Aurelius-Cornelius Celsus (26 B.C.-50 A.D.) whose book De Medicina was printed and widely-distributed in Latin and European languages, including French as late as 1876. De Medicina was published in eight volumes: Four chronicled diseases that could be treated with diet and regimen; the other four focused on diet and surgery. Though Aurelius Celsus was known for his extensive study of medicine, current research including a reliable report in the U.S. National Library of Medicine said, "While Celsus' work is the best account of Roman medicine as practiced in the first century of the Christian era and its influence until the 19th-century, there is controversy as to whether Cornelius actually practiced as a surgeon himself."

Was he, as many now believe, an encyclopedist who collected convincing medical knowledge available at the time, but was neither a practicing physician nor a surgeon? Perhaps so.

Greek physician Rufus of Ephesus (70-110 A.D.) was also among the hierarchy as a learned physician of the age. Details from A History of Medicine by Ralph Major, M.D., once professor and Chairman of Department of History at Kansas University Medical Center. Details of Rufus reveal his history as an anatomist who identified and named various parts of the human body. His book Interrogation of a Patient may be the first ever written on how to take a History from a patient. He stressed the importance of, not only the history of illness, but also family history, social habits and the conditions of the region where the patient lived. Rufus described the symptoms and signs of pneumonia and also wrote about the significance of different characters of pulse. Still in use is his terminology of inflammation—rubor (redness), dolor (pain), tumor (swelling) and color.

Contributions of Arabic medicine cannot be ignored. Arabs translated many of Galen's writings from Greek to Arabic, thus preserving them. SCIplanet, a bilingual science magazine, reported that Muslim physicians proved their ability in all fields of medicine with their mastery in chemistry, biology and dissection. Avicenna (980-1037 A.D.), a Persian philosopher, scientist and physician wrote the Canon of Medicine, still recognized as the standard medical text of the Arabic ancient world.

In England, Oxford University's Medical Science department catalogues John Gaddesden (1280-1360) as a professor at Oxford, a physician to King Edward III, and the leading medical authority of his day. He wrote Rosa Anglica and according to a report in the British Library, Gaddesden said, "The rose excels all flowers so this book excels all treatises on the practice of medicine." Rosa Anglica, the first English textbook of medicine, described cases, signs, and keys to prognosis and cures of illnesses and disease.

The University of Glasgow reported that more than fifty manuscripts containing the texts of England's pre-Renaissance physician John of Aderne (1307-1380) remain today and his texts include hundreds of illustrations. They show procedures, herbs and tools, as well as symbolic representations of abstract concepts, such as pain, all which make the texts more valuable. His best-known work is Practica Chirurgiae, the Practice of Surgery. In it, he detailed the regimen and treatment of fistula-in-ano (anal fistula) and boasted a survival rate of fifty-percent. The Glasgow library referenced John of Aderne as the Father of English Surgery who referred to himself as a master surgeon in his texts. Yet, the library report noted, he is not recognized as such in contemporary records.

More controversial was Paracelsus (1493-1541), Swiss medical doctor and philosopher who provoked controversy and still invokes controversy today, according to an account in the World Research Foundation/ WRF. Briefly a professor at Basel University in Switzerland, his medical works dealt with syphilis and its therapy, illnesses and disease, surgery and the treatment of wounds. He wrote of therapeutic mineral baths in Switzerland, Austria and southern Germany as nature's healers and used metals like mercury, lead, arsenic, iron and copper sulphate in his pharmacopeia. Outspoken and opinionated, WRF noted Paracelsus publicly condemned the medical authority of Avicenna and Galen and flung their writings into the celebration bonfire on St. John's Day 1527.

All in all, even if the Middle Ages were the Dark Ages, physicians and medical texts of the time led to the dawn of the Renaissance.

1301-1600

THE RENAISSANCE
A Sweeping Movement
of Transformational Change

Chapter Twelve

The Rise of the Renaissance

The rise of the Renaissance (1301-1600) was a sweeping movement that inspired transformational changes in philosophy, art, science and religion. Medicine was no exception. The Gutenberg press accelerated printing and publishing which allowed and encouraged diffusion of medical knowledge. Old assumptions were questioned and new thinking flourished in the Renaissance, the French word for rebirth.

It was Greek physician Galen who introduced the concept of medicine as a science and an art, not science alone (in the 2nd-century). And it was a combination of science and art that advanced the understanding of medicine and human anatomy during the Renaissance. Physicians, however, behaved as if it were unthinkable to challenge Galen's anatomy texts that had been accepted and taught for more than nearly two centuries. Among Galen's defenders was famous Parisian physician and educator Jacques Sylvius (1478-1555). Sylvius taught the Belgian physician Andreas Vesalius (1515-1564) who is classified in medical history as a foremost anatomist. Seven volumes of Vesalius' influential book On The Fabric of the Human Body (De Humani Corporis Fabrica Libri Septem) published in 1543 focused on skeleton, muscles, vascular system, nervous system, abdomen, thorax and brain. As a youth, Vesalius had dissected mice, rats and dogs. After his studies with Sylvius, he returned to Belgium to teach the study of the body's internal parts to medical students. The story is, Vesalius dissected bodies of hanged criminals and was knowledgeable based on his studies of such human cadavers. His book is considered to be an amazing study and a masterpiece even today. He was among the many who altered Galen's teachings of anatomy although academia, including his teacher Sylvius, believed Galen's texts on anatomy and physiology to be infallible.

Aware of growing skepticism on Galen's theory of circulation, an Englishman who studied medicine in Italy, William Harvey (1578-1657) further studied circulation of blood through the human body. Based on his research, Harvey published a groundbreaking book in 1628 titled On the Motion of Heart and Blood in Animals. He established the fact that the heart, not the liver, functions as the engine for circulation. Further clarifying Harvey's conclusion is the Source Book of Medical History by Logan Clendening, an American doctor, educator and historian of the 19th-century. So valued is Clendening's Source Book that hard cover copies sell today from $200.00 to $985.00. He quotes Harvey as saying, "Blood passes from the right ventricle of the heart through pulmonary artery to the lungs; from there, through pulmonary vein into the left auricle and to the left ventricle."

In his lifetime, Harvey was unable to explain the connection between veins and arteries, according to a 2018 report in National Geographic History. Four years after Harvey's death, Italian physician Marcello Malpighi (1628-1694) realized the passage that connected arterial and venous systems. Using a microscope, he discovered capillaries connecting the two systems. Thus Malpighi found the missing piece of Harvey's puzzle.

A French army surgeon Ambroise Pare (1510-1590) also ranks as an influential figure in medicine during the Renaissance. Until Pare, the practice to treat a wound was to pour boiling oil into it. In treating war wounds,

Pare introduced cauterization of bleeding arteries, suturing wounds, applying dressings, and in that way, revolutionized wound care.

Academia's opposition to new ideas persisted in the Renaissance and, as Oxford Bibliographies point out, attempts were made to amend the medical knowledge of the ancients. At the same time, classical authors such as Galen, Hippocrates and Avicenna remained important authorities through the 17th-century and physicians, such as Vesalius and Harvey mixed old ideas and new advancements, thus leading the way to more.

While Galen's followers ferociously objected to change, they were eventually forced to accept new findings of physicians from England, Italy and France, among others.

New Science then prevailed in the Renaissance and altered the complex understanding and practice of medicine. In its wake, the supremacy of the Church and monastic teaching shifted, leading to the spread of Protestant Reformation.

Chapter Thirteen

The Reformation

Christianity's dominant role in Europe gave many hospitals around the world the names they have today: St. Mary's...St. Joseph's... St. Teresa's...St. Luke's and more. (In biblical history, St. Luke was a recognized physician, "one who heals."). But when England's reigning King during the Age of the Renaissance, Henry VIII (1491-1547) broke from Catholicism in 1534, the role of the Catholic church in medicine was impacted in a significant way.

Angered by a doctrine of the Catholic church, Henry VIII founded the new Church of England. As Supreme Head of the Church of England, he dissolved or demolished eight-hundred or more Catholic monasteries, reclaiming some as his own. The religious upheaval interrupted the dominance monasteries had held as centers of knowledge with their libraries of medical texts, universities and hospitals.

The Protestant Reformation had begun.

Though he was not a physician, historians credit the German-born theologist Martin Luther (1483-1546) with the start of Protestantism, prior to Henry VIII. Luther, an Austrian monk and a powerful force, used the power of the press to publish his Ninety-Five Theses in 1517. With that, he delivered his teachings to a vast audience and affected university-based medical education. U.K's journal of Christian Medical Fellowship specified Luther's medical recommendations as using apothecaries, physicians and nurses to cure physical ailments when administering to the sick. He proposed fumigation for homes contaminated with the plague and discouraged unnecessary travel and exposure to different places.

While Christianity's ecclesia professed education and rational medicine along with prayer and the will of God, a combination of humanistic medicine, science and advanced understanding of anatomy also strengthened across Europe, disrupting and reforming established institutions, practices and beliefs.

In regard to religion's influence, the importance was, in my mind, freedom of speech and the ability to speak out against the Christian church hierarchy. Prompted by free thinking outside the Church, changes occurred in the culture, democracy, science and religion. Medical treatment and hospitals became more independent and out of the Church's control during the Reformation. Nevertheless, Christianity's legacy of health care in communities remains visible and strong today. My medical education was at St. John's Medical College in Bangalore. I remember Mother Virginia, a nurse, and I remember nuns were not teachers, but they had authority. They were running the place. Later in America, my internship was at Nazareth Hospital in Philadelphia founded in the 19th-century by Sisters of the Holy Family of Nazareth. Without question, the influence of the church extended into contemporary times.

When there is resistance to change, there is also a question: Is transformational change generally good for society and, in this case, medicine? With Reformation embedded in the Age of the Renaissance, is rebirth—French word for Renaissance—appropriate? Perhaps yes, as an interpretation by Oxford Bibliographies accepts that advancements during the Reformation were a catalyst of disruptive change and upheaval, yet beneficial. For one, Henry VIII's Dissolution of Monasteries ended in 1540. Monastic medical libraries had been destroyed, but Abbeys and Monasteries were renewed throughout Europe and eventually, the world. Christianity and Protestantism coexisted. Medical wisdom of the ancients was studied and challenged. Galenic medicine and Galen's findings of anatomy and physiology were amended. Simultaneously, the value of scientific discoveries increased. Textbooks were widely distributed and new studies of anatomy were taught at universities. Essentially, the Bibliographies said, "…a complex mix of dynamic change and traditional healing structures" made the Renaissance and the Reformation "…the most complex and fascinating epoch in the history of medicine." Read on.

There's more. It may be surprising but true that in addition to physicians, major contributions to medicine of the age were made by Renaissance artists.

Chapter Fourteen

The Artists, the Anatomists

Italian artist Leonardo da Vinci (1492-1519) is often classified as the epitome of Renaissance. As a scholar in multiple fields, from sculpture to science, music, mathematics and philosophy, da Vinci is honored for his art and a timeless contribution to medical science. His detailed illustrations of human anatomy, including more than seven-hundred-fifty anatomical sketches of skeleton, muscles, heart, lung, liver, nerves and brain are still valued for scientific accuracy and artistic beauty. To verify the accuracy of his studies, he injected ventricles in the brain with melted wax to assess size and shape. He did the same with sinuses. His most-recognized drawing of Vitruvian Man illustrates a geometric configuration of a nude man with legs apart and arms extended within a superimposed square and a circle.

The accuracy of da Vinci's sketches eclipse that of a foremost anatomist of the Renaissance, Belgian physician Andreas Vesalius. Encyclopedia Brittanica noted that while Leonardo's anatomical drawings are among the most significant achievements of Renaissance science and art, he neither taught nor published them during his lifetime. His illustrations and the Notebook of Leonardo da Vinci were unknown to the outside world for at least two-hundred years after his death. Some historians speculate he did not consider himself a professional in the field of anatomy so he hid his drawings; others say he purposely hid them out of respect for his renown predecessor, Greek physician Galen.

Da Vinci also understood the mechanics of muscle contractions. He recognized that hand movements were controlled muscles below the elbow and muscles above elbow were for strength, like pulling and pushing. An amazing observation was that muscles attach to the ribs so that when they contract, they pull ribs away. This creates a negative pressure, allowing lungs to expand like bellows drawing air. Breathing can then occur with the least amount of energy expenditure, a concept that continues to be taught in medical schools of the current century. An extensive report in the U.S. National Library of

Medicine claims that Leonardo's drawings of the muscular system are "the best" of all his illustrations. Equally valuable are his notes.

Long before Renaissance physician William Harvey's findings on circulation of blood, da Vinci discovered that arteries and veins go through the heart, and the liver does not produce venous blood. In addition to da Vinci, other artists—Great Masters of the Renaissance—are renown for anatomical illustrations:

> • Sculptor and painter Michelangelo (1475-1564) who, at the age of sixteen years, dissected corpses at the convent church of Santo Spirito in Florence. Like da Vinci, Michelangelo observed physicians to learn layers of muscle and bone structures. (Muscarelle Museum, Willilamsburg, Va.)

> • Raphael (1483-1520) earned distinction for his anatomical studies and attention to illustrations of human models. He was one of the first to use women as a model in an age when men were used instead. (Raphael-Sanzio.com)

> • Influenced by the Church, early Renaissance sculptor Donatello (1386-1466) may be best-known for his statue

of St. John the Evangelist. Realistic anatomy of the saint's legs demonstrate Donatello's accurate depiction of the human body. Biographers have said of Donatello's sculptures, "every part of the sculpture's body reflects a perfect and complete understanding of human anatomy." (theartstory.org)

A pantheon of respected and famous artists contributed to the study of medicine in the form of anatomical notes and drawings—adding to the Renaissance history of Reformation, Revelations and Rebirth. Before the end of the age, health care would recognize new births—babies borne with the aid of midwives and, with it, insights devoted to pediatrics.

Chapter Fifteen

With the Woman, With Child

The distinction of writing one of the most significant works in the field of midwifery may belong to the work of German apothecary and physician, Eucharius Rosslin (1470-1526). His Rosegarden for Pregnant Women and Midwives (Der Swangern Frauwen und Hebammen Rosegarten) published in 1513 was accepted worldwide as the authoritative manual for midwives.

The practice of midwifery at the time was connected, but not confined, to the ancient medicine of the Egyptians, Indians and Greco-Romans. It could be said that thanks to Rosslin's Rosegarten, the practice of midwifery blossomed during the Renaissance and early 17th-century as the German version was translated into Czech, Danish, Dutch, English, French, Italian and Latin. Still, childbirth in the age of the Renaissance and on into the 17th-century was a dangerous time. Birth was a private, woman-to-woman process until men entered midwifery, too.

Recommended reading about the contributions and challenges in the history of midwifery—a term meaning with the woman—is a report of Rosslin's Rosegarten in U.S. National Library of Medicine. Other rich resources of midwifery, including the U.K.'s Royal College of Physicians and Oxford Bibliographies, are available online. Here are highlights:

Midwives were expected to bring calm to birthing rooms with darkness, quiet and warmth, as if to recreate the womb. They stood in front of the mother-to-be to receive the baby and cut the umbilical cord. When a newborn was sickly or close to death, midwives were allowed to baptize the baby to cleanse its soul and assure it would go to heaven. They took an oath to promise they would not keep anything from the birth that could be used in witchcraft, a concern that persisted through the ages.

After the Rosegarten manual, other books were published, some cautionary and some highly critical of midwifery as it was practiced in the Renaissance. English physician Thomas Raynalde (1540-1551) published the Byrthe of Mankynde in 1545. His was the first English translation of Der Rosegarten and the first book printed in England with images engraved on copper plates. The images depicted subjects that had not been printed before: the birth chair, birthing room, development of the fetus and its relationship to the uterus. Raynalde's book contained seventeen drawings of children in utero, including an image of conjoined twins. Long before the Victorian Era, Reynaldo reflected a prudish Victorian attitude. "Many might not think it proper," he warned, "to have such matters written in our mother and vulgar language for the detection and discovery by men."

Yet over time, men intervened and the authority of female midwives receded. The rise of the male midwife challenged traditional midwifery, especially in England and France, as noted in the Oxford Bibliographies. Rather than relying on the skills of experienced female midwives to ease the newborn from the birth canal, male attendants turned to the newly-invented forceps. Cutting the umbilical cord also became hotly debated. Trotula, a group of three texts on women's medicine composed by Italian female physician Trota of Salerno (1050-1097), had offered specific instructions for cord cutting: It should be tied and a charm spoken during the cutting, then the cord wrapped "with the string of an instrument that is plucked or bowed." A debate arose over the timing of cutting or clamping the cord. Before or after placental delivery? Which was appropriate?

First written records of cutting before placental delivery were recorded in the 17th-century. Later, British obstetrician Charles White (1728-1813) discredited Trotula's instructions, saying, "The common method of tying and cutting the navel string in the instant the child is born has nothing to plead in its favour but custom."

Over time, the authority of woman-to-woman childbirths diminished due to regulations, lack of midwife's academic education and social attitudes that demeaned them. Men became dominant in the practice of midwifery and male physicians published guide books for midwives. As noted in the Heroine Collective, a U.K. publication, one of the most popular books was Directory for Midwives. It was written by English physician Nicholas Culpepper (1616-1654) who, by his own admission, had never attended a birth. Surpassing Culpepper's directory, was English midwife Jane Sharp (age uncertain). Published in 1671, her Midwives Book: The Whole Art of Midwifery was the first on the subject to be produced by an Englishwoman.

Still, stereotypes of "ignorant" midwives grew. Trained physicians became the choice of the privileged and midwives served in rural or impoverished areas.

Latest statistics show births attended by midwives today is eight-percent in the U.S. and significantly higher in European countries.

By the end of the Renaissance (rebirth), male physicians had become predominant in childbirth. The following century saw the birth of another kind: A spirit of discovery was reborn and would change the practice of medicine forever.

1601-1700, A.D.

SEVENTEENTH-CENTURY
The Spirit of Discovery Spreads

Chapter Sixteen
The Visionaries

A spirit of discovery swiftly spread across Europe, mainly Italy, France, Germany, Belgium and the Netherlands in the 17th-century. An abundance of books and the free-thinking culture of the Renaissance had opened the door to an exchange of ideas, experiments and medical advancements. In a short one-hundred-year span, the invention of a modern microscope, the discovery of bacteria and the birth of microbiology changed medicine forever.

As per Transactions of Leeuwenhoek's Works published in Philosophical Transactions of Royal Society of London, Antonie van Leeuwenhoek (1632-1723), a Dutch scientist, invented a then-advanced microscope. Details in the History of Medicine reveal that Leeuwenhoek identified bacteria in scrapings from his own mouth. He had been interested in developing a microscope from a young age. He experimented with several methods to develop a lens for better magnification and came up with a lens from crushing and polishing ground glass. This improved magnification from what had been fifty times to two-hundred-seventy times. That was the beginning of a modern microscope.

Yet Leeuwenhoek was not the only inventor in the crowded and competitive field of 17th-century visionaries.

Modern historians credit German-Dutch spectacle maker Hans Lipperhey (1570-1610) with inventing the first telescope in the 16th-century and many credit Lipperhey as the inventor of the compound microscope. Lipperhey's Dutch counterpart Zacharias Janssen (1588-1638), also a spectacle maker, is known for creating early models of the telescope and compound microscope. It is believed that he developed his microscope while working with his father Hans Janssen (age unknown). The method for both Lipperhey and Janssen was to use two lenses in a tube to create magnification. Even earlier, Italian inventors including Galileo (1564-1642) are noted for inventing the telescope. Yet, many historians agree that Galileo was most likely aware of Lipperhey's invention of the telescope before he developed his own, said Florida State University's Pioneers in Optics report.

A noticeable distinction between the work of Galileo and Lipperhey is that Galileo focused on distant objects, like stars and planets, while Lipperhey focused on magnification of the small objects. His invention was a continuation from a telescope to a powerful microscope. There is still uncertainty about who invented what and when. In fact, a prominent Dutch diplomat accused Lipperhey of stealing his ideas from Janssen and Janssen's father.

According to Pioneers in Optics, "Lipperhey is at least the first to describe a telescope in writing." But ultimately, credit for developing the modern microscope most likely belongs to Leeuwenhoek.

In the confusion and controversy of who first created the microscope, the pioneering Leeuwenhoek's work was sidelined and given scant credit at the time. Being a scientist, not a physician, Leeuwenhoek supposedly did not realize the significance of his discovery of bacteria and the effect of bacteria was not realized until two-hundred years later when famed French biologist Louis Pasteur (1822-1895) discovered microbes. Leeuwenhoek advanced his work and went on to identify red blood cells, yeast and sperms. Another of Leeuwenhoek's many contributions was discovering capillaries between arteries and veins. He confirmed the findings of Marcello Malpighi, a16th-century Italian anatomy professor who had discovered that capillaries were the missing link between arteries and veins in British physician William Harvey's discovery of circulation (referenced in Chapter Twelve).

The list of 17th-century medical visionaries, methods of diagnoses, treatment of afflictions and monumental change in the practice of medicine continued far into the following centuries, even as advancements continued to evolve.

Chapter Seventeen

Inventions, Advancements and a Few Flops

The 17th-century goes down in history as a time of inventions and procedures that revolutionized medicine. While many pioneers in medicine are renown for advancements and eradication of deadly diseases, such as measles, others are known for experiments that went wrong.

One of the best-known and still-honored pioneers of the time is Thomas Sydenham (1624-1689). Classified as the English Hippocrates, Sydenham was a renown clinical observer. His knowledge and colorful clinical descriptions are unparalleled even today. His still-famous book, The Process of Healing (Processus Integri), was published posthumously with a mere twenty copies in 1692. Other significant Sydenham texts were published and translated in his lifetime, yet his rise to fame as the English equivalent of

Hippocrates was also posthumous. Today, Sydenham's general philosophy of diseases and treatment is verified in scholarly texts, such as The History of Medicine. His Process of Healing was eventually republished and latently became a major reference text for practitioners for more than a century.

The early symptoms of measles, an infection seen predominantly in children, were vividly described by Sydenham. He explained how the rash starts behind the ear on the first day and then spreads all over the patient's face by fifth day. Sydenham went on to describe how healing began, starting from the sixth day, if no complications, such as pneumonia or meningitis occurred. He recommended treatments to control fever and cough and also warned of potential long-term complications.

In the pre-vaccine age, America's Center for Disease Control/CDC reports that nearly all children got measles by the time they were fifteen-years old. Measles epidemics were global and in the U.S. alone, the CDC estimated three to four million people were infected each year. As many as five-hundred of the affected died, thousands were hospitalized and thousands suffered encephalitis (swelling of the brain) caused by measles. A case of measles is rarely seen in modern medicine because of a vaccine developed in the U.S. in 1963 by John Franklin Enders (1897-1985), an American biomedical scientist and Nobel Laureate. The mortality rate has improved significantly since the introduction of vaccines, though it remains high in developing countries.

In addition to measles, Sydenham's colorful way of describing symptoms in a variety of afflictions has proven to be an effective way—perhaps the best way—to teach students. His impressive descriptions of diseases are taught in medical schools today and cited in JCR: Journal of Clinical Rheumatology, among other publications. My personal exposure to Sydenham was as a young medical student. I remember learning about St. Vitus dance, a manifestation of rheumatic fever, based on Sydenham's vivid description. His description of a peculiar convulsion and gesticulations as a dance still sticks in my mind.

Among his most useful descriptions is how gout starts and progresses. He identified gout as a disease affecting older men and referenced heredity and red wine as factors in the causes of gout. The condition usually starts in the big toe and is extremely painful, he explained. He went on to reveal complications and recommended treatment of gout. South Africa's Nature Life notes that gout, a type of arthritis is on the rise, particularly in America. Historically in all countries, gout afflicted famous names you know, from King Henry VIII to German composer Beethoven; American statesman Benjamin Franklin; British writer Charles Dickens; Italy's tenor Luciano Pavarotti and artist Leonardo da Vinci and this century's North Korean Kim Jong-Un who, Nature Life said, "...apparently has a penchant for Swiss Emmental cheese and red wine."

In addition to Sydenham, other colorful stories are tied to the 17th-century—three are bloody tales. One tells of the first attempt of blood transfusion in1665 by an English physician Richard Lower (1631-1691). He demonstrated a dog-to-dog transfusion in front of an audience at a Royal Society meeting. Unexpectedly, the donor dog died but the recipient dog survived. Then in 1667, a prominent French physician Jean-Baptiste Denys (1643-1704) faced a situation of excessive bleeding in a boy that had resulted from a bloodletting procedure. Kat Escher, writing for Smithsonian magazine, said Denys performed the first documented blood transfusion on the fifteen-year-old boy. Because of the dire emergency, Dynes transfused the boy with a half pint of lamb's blood.

"Somehow," Escher wrote in the Smithsonian, "the boy survived." But Dynes' continued procedures were botched. He repeated the procedure with lamb's blood until a patient died following the transfusion. Dynes was formally charged with murder. He was acquitted, but a law to ban transfusions was passed in France. The ban lasted until 1818 when the first human-to-human transfusion was successfully carried out, more than one-hundred years after Jean-Baptiste Denys died. Even then, the safety of transfusions was established far into the future, only after the 1901 discovery of blood grouping by an Austrian physician Karl Landsteiner (1868-1943) and cross-matching technique in early 1907 by Czech doctor Jan Jansky (1873-1921).

In addition to transfusions, bleeding from war wounds and surgery continued to present a bloody challenge. In fact, the U.K.'s Historic Coventry report was emphatic in saying, "Surgery was gruesome." Though surgery was recorded in ancient Greek, Indian and Egyptian texts, it was neither a popular nor successful field during the Middle Ages and through the 17th-century. The main reasons were pain, lack of anesthetic agents and an extremely high incidence of infection and death following surgery. Surgical instruments were unclean, some were rusty, and surgeons operated in their every-day clothes, the Historic Coventry said. No wonder surgeons were identified as barbers in England.They were addressed as mister or as barber-surgeons while other physicians were addressed as doctor.

To stop bleeding in war wounds, surgeons routinely poured boiling oil into the wound to cauterize blood vessels which often made the wounds worse. While French army surgeon Ambroise Pare (d. 1590) pioneered in battlefield medicine and treatment of wounds during the Renaissance, his techniques included cauterization of bleeders and suturing of wounds. It was not until the 19th-century that anesthesia was introduced and surgery became attractive to physicians.

Still, while illness and disease continued to plague humans, medicine was on the brink of brilliant new discoveries in the century ahead.

1701-1800, A.D.

THE EIGHTEENTH-CENTURY
An Impact on M edicine for All Time

Chapter Eighteen

Vaccination

Smallpox was a scourge that battered the human race at least from the Roman era or before, resulting in significant mortality and severe disfigurement among those who survived. Miraculously, 18th-century discoveries eradicated smallpox around the globe and the age of preventive medicine began. Vaccination and other protections against diseases were developed by physicians and, unexpectedly, by a non-physician. A lady.

Lady Mary Montagu (1689-1762), an English aristocrat, settled in Turkey for a time as the wife of Edward Wortley Montagu (1678-1761), British Ambassador to the Ottoman Empire. In Turkey, Lady Mary noticed the skin of the locals was unscarred from smallpox. At the time, the only known treatment for the deadly pox was isolating victims to prevent contagion. But Lady Mary's investigation of unscarred survivors led to a status celebrated today with a glaring headline in a recent issue of Time magazine: How One Daring Woman Introduced the Idea of Smallpox Inoculation to England.

Time's writer Thomas Hager claims that Lady Mary "…laid the groundwork for what today we would call inoculation and the eventual eradication of the disease." But, of course, there was controversy. Here's what happened:

Written notes from the time indicate that Turkish physicians had developed a method where postulant material from a smallpox patient was rubbed into a scratch on a healthy person. This did not prevent smallpox in the person, but the attack was mild. Lady Mary herself had suffered through smallpox, known as "the speckled monster," a disease that was the deadliest on earth, Hager wrote in Time. In a 1717 letter, Lady Mary spread news of a phenomenon she witnessed in Turkey. "Commonly, as many as sixteen people gather to be treated," she said. "They make parties for this purpose." Then "…an old woman comes with a nut-shell full of the matter of smallpox. With something that may have been a large needle, scratching the skin, then the puss from someone who had smallpox, the old woman puts into the vein as much matter as can lie upon the head of her needle."

Lady Mary experimented by trying the technique on her two daughters and both developed only a mild form of smallpox. Upon returning to England, her attempt to popularize the process was ineffective, actually banned. What she had done remained dormant and was overshadowed by Edward Jenner (1749-1823), a country doctor in England. Jenner observed that dairy workers who had contracted cowpox, a viral disease on cows' udders, would then have only a mild form of smallpox. He took material from an eruption in the hand of a milkmaid who was afflicted with cowpox and injected it to an eight-year-old boy. The boy developed cowpox and recovered. Jenner then exposed the child to conventional smallpox and the boy did not develop smallpox.

Jenner's experiment led to development of smallpox vaccine in 1798. Now, two-hundred years later, smallpox is wiped out from the earth. His discovery was the beginning of vaccination to prevent communicable diseases. As a result, many are eradicated from the world.

Science gives Jenner credit for developing the smallpox vaccination, but as it was with discoveries in the 17th-century, credit was given to one while it may have belonged to another. Some accounts say Lady Mary applied secretions directly to the skin and what Jenner did was injections. Questions remain:

- Is it not true that credit should also be given to Lady Mary who dared to test the concept on her own children?

- Did Lady Mary use a needle as some recent reports imply?

- Is it possible that the country doctor Jenner got the ideas from her?

Hager's conclusion in Time magazine is that Lady Mary's great achievement remained little-known until recent years. He quotes British scientist Sir Francis Galton (1822-1911) who said, "'In science, the credit goes to the one who convinces the world, not to whom the idea first occurs."

What matters, though, is that smallpox is gone. And it matters that discoveries did not end with Jenner and Lady Mary. Other notable physicians, scientists, educators, and anatomists continued to define medicine of the 18th-century and impact the future of medicine for all time.

Chapter Nineteen

Lady With the Lamp and Medicine Worldwide

Throughout medical history, trailblazing initiatives were slow to be adopted. Still, life-altering discoveries quickly sprang from the 19th-century's one-hundred year span and are recognized as a foundation for modern medicine. One of the brightest stars to emerge in the century was a legendary British nurse whose name you know. Nightingale.

So well remembered is nurse Florence Nightingale (1820-1910) that the year 2020 was declared International Year of Nurses, the two-hundredth anniversary of Nightingale's birth. The professional journal Nurse marked the milestone with a featured story and a bold headline: Imagine if Florence Nightingale Lived Today.

A 21st-century practitioner Barbara Dossey, Ph.D RN says emphatically that if nurse Nightingale lived now she would see her initiatives are as relevant in today's world as they were in her time. Dossey, International Coordinator of the Nightingale Institute for Global Health, quotes from Nightingale's personal diary that predicted it would take as many as one-hundred-fifty years to see the kind of nursing Nightingale envisioned. How true it is. Gradually over time, her efforts to train and educate have elevated the status of nursing to the level of a noble profession worldwide. Yet Nightingale's path to world fame as a nurse was not without challenges.

While she was young, she felt a call from God to devote her life to others. She chose to become a nurse, but as an English lady born into an aristocracy, her family disapproved of the idea. The nursing profession was not viewed with high esteem in an elite society at the time. Against objections, she chose nursing as her vocation and volunteered to travel to Turkey to care for soldiers wounded in the deadly Crimean War of 1853 to 1856.

Appalled by the casualty count and the care wounded soldiers received, nurse Nightingale worked, tirelessly it is said, to improve the quality of medical care and prevent the spread of infection to wounds with hygiene and cleanliness. At night, she was known to walk in hospital wards to monitor patients while carrying a Turkish lantern in her hand, hence earning the name The Lady with the Lamp.

When she returned to England, she focused her attention on advancing the quality of education for nurses. In 1860, she used her own funds to establish the world's first professional nursing school at St. Thomas Hospital in London. Now part of King's College London, nursing graduates take the Nightingale Pledge, so named in her honor. Long before United Nations founded the World Health Organization in 1948, Nightingale had traveled the globe to improve nursing care and rural health. Thus nurses' professional organizations as well as universities offer continuing education opportunities, such as Florence Nightingale: Connecting Her Legacy with Local-to-Global Health Today.

Personally, as a physician who practiced medicine and worked with nurses for over fifty years, I can say physicians often get the credit for diagnoses and treatment, but nurses are the ones who complete the delivery of care. Physicians are often paternalistic and for one reason or another do not have the time or patience to explain treatments or educate the patient. Nurses bridge that gap in addition to their regular nursing duties and staying up-to-date with continued education.

Biographies of Nightingale's life and history are abundant and she alone published as many as two-hundred books, pamphlets and articles. Her Notes on Nursing covered basic care for nurses to provide and the book became a canon of nursing. Beyond teaching nursing care, she encouraged personal hygiene, nutrition, exercise and in the Nightingale Pledge, faithfulness and purity. She was also an expert statistician. With evidence from graphs and charts she created, she demonstrated the rate of soldier's mortality beyond the battlefield and convinced officials of shortcomings in their care. By promoting social reforms and the need for women's education and employment, she may be thought of as the first to start the feminist movement.

The Lady With the Lamp, a beacon of hope, still shines as do other contributors to the scientific and medical pantheon of the time. Imagine if they lived today what they would see:

- The concept of British naturalist Charles Darwin (1809-1884) is still studied as the foundation for the theory of evolution and natural selection, even though Darwin't Origin of Species was published in 1859.

- Austrian monk Gregor Mendel (1822-1884) retains the title Father of Modern

Genetics for his discovery while growing peas in the monastic garden.

• British doctor John Snow (1813-1858) proved the deadly disease of cholera spread by drinking contaminated water. Cholera has been controlled, not ended, and still plagues the poor in third-world nations.

• Guido Baccelli (1832-1916), an Italian physician, is credited for pioneering intravenous therapy in the late 1890s. Further developed in the 1930s and widely available in the 1950s, Baccelli had led the way to intravenous medicine today.

• A "moral" movement fostered by French physician Philippe Pinel (1745-1826) and U.S. reformer Dorothy Dix (1802-1887) resulted in more humane and compassionate treatment for the mentally ill and a changed perception of psychiatric patients today.

Clearly, European doctors and scientists contributed to the dawn of preventive medicine in the 19th-century and opened a gateway to global medicine of the future. Though only a small number of American practitioners made notable discoveries, America and other countries came on strong in the following century.

1801-1900, A.D.

NINETEENTH-CENTURY
The Dawn of Preventive Medicine

Chapter Twenty

Prevention, Invention, Innovation

The 19th-century heralded the dawn of modern medicine and gave birth to the foundation for detecting bacterial infection. It saw the invention of the stethoscope, a symbol of the medical profession. It also introduced anesthesia during surgery and the Nightingale who revolutionized the nursing profession. Eminent and ambitious medical practitioners of the time wrote profusely and spread their knowledge of diseases and treatments.

The concept of preventive medicine had begun.

Until the 19th-century, there was no valid way to analyze breath sounds and heart sounds. Physicians had relied on detailed history and observation of external signs for diagnoses. The usual practice was for doctors to hold an ear close to the chest to listen to the sounds. That changed with the innovation of

French physician Rene Laennec (1781-1826). As the story goes, Laennec was called to see a patient who had chest problems. When he arrived at the house, he noticed his patient was a young lady who was considerably obese. He was embarrassed to put his ear close her chest. He then remembered an incident he had observed on the street where a gathering of boys played with what appeared to be a hollow tube. One set of boys would scratch one end of the tube and the sound was channeled to boys listening at the other end.

Laennec decided to try the technique of transferring sound by rolling a paper and placing one end on the lady's chest and the other close to his ear. Laennec, the physician, was also a musician attuned to sound and, to his amazement, he heard the heart and breath sounds through the paper roll. He experimented further to perfect the transmission of sound through hollow tubes. After a series of trials, he came up with two rubber tubes attached to a flat metal piece for the chest and two knobs for the ears. With that, he could hear the heart and breath sounds with clarity. He named the tool a stethoscope (from Greek word stethos for chest and scope to observe).

Laennec's innovation was the beginning of auscultation which became an integral part of physical examination by physicians. Eventually the stethoscope replaced the Aesculapian staff with the image of a snake around it as the symbol of the medical profession.

In earlier centuries, physicians had tried to develop new methodologies and attempts to reduce the pain of surgery was among them. Herbal medicines and opium had been tried without any effect. In the middle of the 19th-century, an American dentist from Boston, Massachusetts, Horace Wells (1815-1848), successfully used nitrous oxide (laughing gas) to dull pain. A publication of the American Society of Anesthesiologists/ASA, credits Wells with showing "great courage in undergoing the extraction of his own tooth under nitrous oxide to prove its effectiveness and verify its analgesic properties." The tooth was extracted by a colleague and dentist, also based in Boston, John M. Riggs (1811-1885). Riggs was later honored for his treatment of periodontal disease alveolar pyorrhea (neglected gingivitis and poor oral hygiene), a condition named Riggs' disease.

The laughing gas was successful at reducing pain in dental procedures, but failed in its use during surgery. And Wells led a failed attempt to convince the medical and dental professions of the efficacy of nitrous oxide, said the ASA report.

The quest to find other methods of pain control continued throughout the century. Another American dentist, W.T. Morgan (1819-1868) used ether for a painless tooth extraction. Before Morgan, it is believed that American physician Crawford Williamson Long (1815-1878) was first to discover ether as an anesthetic. In the New Georgia Encyclopedia, medical historian M. Leslie Madden wrote that Long, a Georgia physician, successfully used the gas when he removed a tumor from the neck of a young man. He performed more surgeries using ether, but did not publish his findings, perhaps because doctors were skeptical and critics accused Long of practicing witchcraft. Others believed he was disturbing the natural order of things and that pain was God's way of cleansing the soul, the New Georgia Encyclopedia said. Also, ether had several side effects including an unpredictable length of its effect.

Sir James Young Simpson (1811-1870), a Scottish physician, experimented with several chemicals and eventually came upon chloroform. It was being used in small doses for other conditions, though not for surgery. A report by the Royal College of Physicians of Edinburgh tells that Simpson and two assistants tested chloroform by inhaling and they "quickly fell to the ground." With further attempts, Simpson found that liquid chloroform evaporated quickly and was easy to administer and effective during surgery. Chloroform continued to be used for anesthesia for years before current-day medications were invented.

Previously, bacteria had been identified with a microscope by Dutch scientist Antonie Leeuwenhoek in the 17th-century. But it was 19th-century French biologist Louis Pasteur (1822-1895) who earns credit for perfecting the technique of culturing and staining the bacteria. This paved the way for clinical use bacteriology in identifying infectious diseases. Much has been written about the renown Pasteur and the consensus is that Pasteur supported the germ theory which became the foundation of bacteriology. He also discovered that microorganisms were responsible for spoiling beverages like alcohol and milk and he explained the process of fermentation. Pasteur proved that when heated above a certain temperature, the bacteria are killed and when cooled they are safe for consumption—pasteurized—as milk is today before it is brought to market.

An added discovery of the great scientist Pasteur was a vaccine for rabies, an infection which even today is fatal if untreated. Pasteur injected a rabbit with an extract from the spinal cord of a rabid dog and the rabbit developed rabies. He injected the material from this rabbit to successive rabbits. The infection became less virulent after each attempt. He then injected a dog with spinal cord substance, exposing the dog to rabies, but the dog did not develop the disease. A boy named Joseph Meister (1876-1940) was bitten several times by a rabid dog and was sure to develop rabies. Pasteur gave thirteen injections to the abdominal wall of the boy and the child, miraculously, did not develop rabies. That was the birth of vaccine for rabies and the young Meister lived more than sixty years.

Subsequent studies by Pasteur led to development of vaccine for chicken cholera, a highly contagious and lethal disease in poultry yards, and for anthrax, a common affliction in domestic and wild animals around the world. He also developed a cellular egg production method to preserve healthy silkworm eggs—important because silkworms produce silk threads and, genetically modified by scientists in Japan, secrete collagen. In China, dead silkworm bodies produce a medicine for human conditions, such as flatulence and body spasms. Plus, silkworms are a popular and healthy snack in some countries, according to The Guardian, an environmentally friendly network. In China and Vietnam, silkworms are fried; In Korea, silkworms are seasoned and boiled.

The list of preventive medical discoveries did not stop with Pasteur. The advancement of preventive medicine throughout the 19th-century marched on and on.

Chapter Twenty-One
Preventitive Medicine Marches On

Founded on science, research and determination to gain knowledge, medical breakthroughs of the 19th-century were widely communicated and spread around the globe. Few would equal achievements of the century's acclaimed French biologist Louis Pasteur, but other ingenious discoveries in the field of medicine were undeniable.

A contemporary of Pasteur, German physician and microbiologist Heinrich Hermann Robert Koch (1843-1910), identified tuberculosis bacteria from the sputum of a patient. He then developed the technique to stain the bacteria, the cause of illness and death from tuberculosis (called consumption). Koch won the Nobel Prize for his work in 1905, five years before his death at age sixty-seven.

Another Nobel laureate of the era was Paul Ehrlich (1854-1915), a German-born physician and bacteriologist most famous for the "magic bullet" concept. Like a gun firing a bullet to a target, his theory was to inject a chemical to aim at the organism, such as bacteria, the cause of the disease. Ehrlich proved his theory by injecting arsenic to treat syphilis. This was the beginning of chemotherapy. His research also led to the discovery of the immune system. When the body is attacked by a pathogen (antigen), the body responds by developing antibodies to fight the invading agent. This was the beginning of the field of immunology.

In 1908, Ehrlich was awarded the Nobel Prize in Physiology, an honor shared with Russian biologist Elie Metchnikoff (1845-1916), the Science History Institute of Philadelphia reminds its readers. The distinction between Ehrlich and Metchnikoff was their paths to understanding the immune response. Ehrlich, the institute noted, presented a chemical theory to explain the formation of antitoxins or antibodies to fight toxins released by bacteria. Metchnikoff studied the role of white corpuscles in destroying bacteria themselves. The Nobel committee apparently reached a consensus and agreed that both explanations of the immune system were necessary.

These concepts are relevant in today's cancer treatment and efforts to fight the worldwide grip of the deadly Corona virus in the year 2020 (and beyond). Attempts to personalize cancer treatment by developing a drug to target the specific cancer cell is a form of what Ehrlich himself labelled the magic bullet theory. Ehrlich's contributions also extend to hematology. He developed a method for staining blood cells with dyes and identified different cells like red, white lymphocytes in the blood.

Ehrlich is considered the Father of Chemotherapy. The significance of his contributions in bacteriology, immunology, chemotherapy and hematology have extended beyond his lifetime and remain relevant in medicine today, according to scholarly journals. Still, it is my personal opinion that Ehrlich's trail-blazing contributions do not get enough recognition. When I read about these fields of medicine, I find very little is written about Ehrlich and his impact on what is happening today with chemotherapy and immunology. Looking back, I see his discoveries are indeed relevant now and should be widely recognized. A friend and colleague of mine agrees that hardly anyone in medicine talks about Ehrlich. Somehow, it is Koch who is given more importance.

Nevertheless, 19th-century breakthroughs are profound and far-reaching well into the 21st-century. The Royal College of

Physicians of Edinburgh considers the brilliant contributions of Scottish physician Sir James Young Simpson astounding. In 1869, one year before his death, Simpson took up a final cause by promoting the rights of women to enter the medical field. According to the Royal College, he encouraged women to "attend the class of any professor who is willing to teach them." Simpson's futuristic advice supports the advance of female physicians and indirectly links to the nursing profession and a singular Nurse Nightingale of the 19th-century.

1901-2000, A.D.

TWENTIETH-CENTURY
European Influence Lessens
American Influence Grows

Chapter Twenty-Two
A Miracle Drug
and Medical Pioneers

Achievements of the 18th-century proved that the pace of medical discoveries had accelerated. In a short span of time, not only was a life-saving vaccine created, but pioneering physicians continued to develop treatments to impact life and death, then and now.

Among the leaders was an English botanist and physician, William Withering (1741-1799), who developed an extract from Foxglove, a colorful plant that grew like a weed in England, and a miracle drug ensued. Withering created a drug that is widely used today and, according to History of Science journal, it is still tied to "one physician and one beautiful wild flower."

When given to patients with leg swelling from heart failure, Withering found that the patient showed significant improvement. His medicine was composed, the journal said, of an herbal mixture, a "long-kept secret by an old woman in Shropshire." The woman sometimes made cures after traditional methods had failed. The mixture combined a variety of herbs, but Withering perceived that the active herb was Foxglove.

His clinical experience with the purple Foxglove was detailed in a paper published in 1775. In it, he discussed more than one-hundred patients who were treated with the medicinal drug. Of those, one-hundred-one patients with congestive heart failure experienced relief, the journal reported. The active ingredient in Foxglove is digitalis, Latin name for the plant, Digitalis purpurea. Digoxin is a mainstay treatment of heart failure today.

In the same century, a noted educator and professor of anatomy at Padua School of medicine in Padua, Italy, Giovanni Battista Morgagni (1682-1771) recorded detailed descriptions of abnormal physical signs observed in his patients during their lives. Throughout his fifty-two-year university tenure, he performed autopsies in patients and attempted to correlate abnormal physical findings with pathological findings in autopsy. With that, Morgagni validated clinical findings and eventually earned the title Father of Modern Anatomy and Pathology. His book On the Seats and Causes of Diseases (De Sed-

ibus et Causis Morborum per Anatomen Ind-
agitis) published in 1761 is classified by Brittanica as Morgagni's greatest work, a valuable
source for practitioners to assess the status of
internal organs by external clinical signs.

By means of observation, an innovative
diagnostic tool was made by Leopold Auenbrugger (1722-1809), an Austrian physician
who emerged as a medical pioneer of the century. Auenbrugger had worked in his father's
tavern as a young boy. He had noticed his father tapped the wine barrels to assess the level
of wine inside: a dull sound indicated a full
wine level; a hollow sound indicated empty.
When examining patients with fluid in the
lung or air in the lining of lung, Auenbrugger
applied this technique of placing one hand
flat on the chest and tapping with the middle
finger from the other hand. He then could de-
cipher the consistency of the structure under-
neath, solid or air. This was the beginning of
the diagnostic technique of percussion used
by physicians even today. The technique is
helpful in diagnosing pneumonia, pneumo-
thorax, margins of heart, lung, liver, and other organs.

All in all, the 18th-century represented
an aggressive pace of medical discoveries and
signaled the entrance to even more monumental treatment methods in the years ahead.

Chapter Twenty-Three

Tests and Diagnosis

America led the march to develop multiple investigatory techniques to facilitate and improve the accuracy of diagnosis during the 20th-century. It was a time when the European influence in medicine was lessening and the American influence was increasing. Money began to flow in America.

The United States government, universities, private enterprise, philanthropic donors and the prominent National Institute of Science established in 1996 poured money into medical research. That's likely the reason America took center stage. Remarkable discoveries of previous centuries had laid the groundwork for global medicine but were further advanced, perfected and made more useful in the 1900s. Still, pioneers of the 17th- through 19th-centuries should not be overlooked.

Invention of X-Rays toward the end of the 19th-century was a major step in the use of tests for diagnosis. From plain X-Rays, new methods of fluoroscopic examinations and use of barium to provide contrast helped the impact of X-Rays even further. By the 1960s, the CT scan was introduced. This used X-Rays to create images of internal organs and help detect tumors or abnormal swellings or bleeding internally. A significant advantage was differentiating mass bleeding in the brain. Until then, diagnoses were based on clinical signs and often guess work, sometimes with disastrous outcomes.

In the 1970s, the MRI was introduced. Here radio-frequency pulse was used in a magnetic field to create images of internal organs. This gave more detailed images and showed even small pathologies, especially in soft tissues. The MRI took more time and expense, but was more effective in diagnosis. These advanced X-Ray technologies improved diagnosis of cancer, small fractures and small bleedings.

Unfortunately, liberal use of the tests resulted in more costs and, in my assessment, overuse. A classic example is the use of tests for patients with back pain when we know that a bulging disc is common over the age of fifty and ordering these tests without clinical suspicion of neurological damage can result in unnecessary and expensive treatments.

Blood Count (CBC) is extremely helpful in a wide range of clinical situations, such as bleeding, anemia and cancer. German physiologist of the 19th-century, Karl von Vierordt (1818-1884), developed a method to count the number of blood cells in one millimeter of blood in a capillary tube and view it under a microscope. Other pioneers of the previous era were German-born Nobel Laureate Paul Ehrlich and Dimitri Romanowsky (1861-1921). They developed a technique to separate and count red and white blood cells. A later method developed in the 1920s to count cells automatically made blood count easier. Since several salts and minerals are present in the blood, excess or deficiency of elements like sodium, potassium bicarbonate can cause serious medical complications, especially in an ICU setting. In 1903, Svante Arrhenius (1859-1927), a Swedish physicist and chemist, won the Nobel prize by developing a technique for separating and measuring levels of these elements in the blood. This was a major step in an acute care setting.

As early as 1769, cholesterol in blood was identified by French physician Francois Poulletier de la Salle (1719-1788). By 1955, American scientist John William Gofman

(1918-2007), a professor at University of California Berkeley, advanced the understanding of cholesterol by inventing an ultracentrifuge technique to separate different types of cholesterol in plasma, thus discovering the role of LDL and HDL in heart disease.

Clergyman Stephen Hales (1677-1761) of England, a Doctor of Divinity, not a medical doctor, and French physiologist Claude Bernard (1813-1878) experimented with catheterization techniques, but it was Werner Forssmann (1904-1979), a physician from Germany, who successfully demonstrated the procedure in 1929. He used his own body by inserting a catheter in his arm and threading it to the heart under fluoroscopic guidance. Now catheterization can be done for many organs, including the brain. Certain procedures, such as removing clots and correcting aneurisms can be done through these catheters. Forssmann shared the 1956 Nobel Prize in physiology with Americans Andre Frederic Cournand (1895-1988) and Dickinson W. Richards (1895-1973).

Cardiac catheterization was a major step in diagnosing heart diseases. The procedure involves inserting a catheter into an artery in the groin or arm and threading it to the heart and then injecting a dye. This demonstrates blood vessels around the heart showing the amount of blockage or malfunction of heart valves, if any. Based on this procedure, a decision can be made on whether the blocked artery needs a stent to keep it open or if bypass surgery is necessary.

The first successful coronary bypass surgery was performed in 1960 at the Albert Einstein College of Medicine by New York physician Robert Hans Goetz (1910-2000), according to a Surgical Heritage report from Mayo Clinic, Rochester, Minnesota. "The name of Goetz, however, means very little if anything, to most surgeons," said the clinic's cardiovascular surgeon Igor Konstantinov. "Only a few know the fact that Goetz was first to successfully perform the surgery."

The list goes on.

Modern history reports that an instrument to look inside hollow organs originated by ancient Greeks and Romans. However, the first documented use of endoscopic procedures were in 1806 by German doctor Philipp Bozzini (1773-1809). It was constructed of a tube before Irish surgeon and urologist Francis Cruise (1834-1912) improved the endoscope by adding light and examining bladder, throat and colon and using it successfully in 1865. In the 1940s, Nobel laureates Cournand and Richards used the instrument for clinical purposes.

Tests and techniques proved to facilitate and improve the accuracy of diagnoses in the 20th-century, often referred to as the American Century of Medicine. Cutting-edge discoveries of the era continued at a rapid pace and progressed to the science of Wonder Drugs.

Chapter Twenty-Four
Transplants: the Age of Replacement Organs

A legend in the Catholic church is that 4th-century Saint Damian and Saint Cosmos transplanted a leg of a diseased Ethiopian to Deacon Justinian who lost a leg due to gangrene. Whatever may be the authenticity of this story or miracle, transplanting organs was a dream for ages.

Sushruta, an Indian surgeon from 1st-century B.C., is reported to have done skin grafts. In 1596, an Italian surgeon Gaspare Tagliacozzi (1545-1599) performed a skin graft and is ranked as a pioneer of plastic and reconstructive surgery. In 1883, Swedish surgeon Theodor Kocher (1841-1917) implanted thyroid tissue in a patient who underwent total removal of the thyroid gland for a goiter. Apparently, this was successful since Kocher was awarded the 1909 Nobel Prize for his work on the thyroid gland.

In the 18th- and 19th-century, several experimental transplants in animals and humans were attempted. Many involved transplanting smaller organs like testicles, ovaries and adrenals. Success of these experiments was short lived.

In 1954, a breakthrough happened when the first successful human-to-human kidney transplant was performed. American surgeon Joseph Edward Murray (1919-2012) of Brigham and Women's Hospital in Boston successfully transplanted a kidney from a human donor to the donor's identical twin brother. The recipient, according to a report from transplantliving.org, went on to live an active normal life, dying eight years later from causes unrelated to the transplant. The kidney transplant opened the door for more, although rejection of a transplanted organ brought a major challenge. The eventual discovery of Cyclosporine helped resolve the problem to a great extent. Now kidney transplants from live and cadaver donors have since become quite common.

The possibility of heart transplant was the dream for people in medicine and in the 20th-century, heart transplant surgery was on the horizon. In 1963, James D. Hardy (1918-2003), a United States surgeon, performed the world's first lung transplant at University of Mississippi Medical Center in Jackson. The patient John Russell, a convict in the Mississippi state penitentiary, lived for eighteen days. Hardy later transplanted a heart from a chimpanzee to a human. The heartbeat lasted only for one hour.

In 1967, South African cardiac surgeon Christiaan Barnard (1922-2001) won acclaim for performing the first human-to-human heart transplant to Louis Washkansky (1913-1967) at Groote Schuur Hospital in Cape Town. Washkansky's heart beat normally, but without anti-rejection drugs, he died of pneumonia within eighteen days, reported History online. History also reported the technique Barnard employed had been initially developed by a group of American researchers in the 1950s and the first successful heart transplant—in a dog—was achieved in 1958 by surgeon Norman Shumway (1923-2006) at Stanford University School of Medicine. Stanford also claimed Shumway performed the first successful human heart transplant in the United States in 1968, one year after Barnard's achievement in South Africa.

The journal Modern Health Care gives the same 1968 distinction of performing the first successful heart transplant to Denton Cooley (1920-2016), founder of the Texas Heart Institute. He first started with valve replacements. He then developed the first heart-lung machine which can temporarily bypass circulation from the heart while performing surgery. This led to successful heart transplants. His prolonged feud with his mentor Michael DeBakey (1908-2008) a Lebanese-American cardiac surgeon in Texas, made interesting news stories during the 1970s. In his own words, Cooley told the U.S. National Library: "My associates and I became the first surgeons in Houston to use a pump oxygenator. Because this breakthrough was accomplished without Dr. DeBakey's knowledge or participation, it marked the beginning of rivalry." The rift lasted forty years.

Gradually, the success rate of transplants improved with better post-operative care and methods to fight rejection with drugs like Cyclosporine. That prompted more transplants, such as liver, lung, pancreas and other organs, including the human face in 2005. Transplant procedures have become highly organized with a transplant registry where names of eligible recipients for each organ are entered. Any possible donor, usually an accident victim, is matched with a potential recipient on the registry. The system then procures the organ and transfers it to the recipient's hospital to transplant as quickly as possible. There is also a program to encourage people to sign for organ donor ship, a boon for medical science.

The first reported joint replacement was in 1891 by Themistocles Gluck (1853-1942). Gluck, a German physician and surgeon created an artificial hip made from ivory in Berlin in 1890. Many other attempts to replace hip joints followed in the 1950s. In the United States, American orthopedic surgeon Austin Moore (1899-1963) ushered in the era of prosthetic replacements in 1940 by successfully performing a partial hip replacement which is named after him. British orthopedic surgeon Sir John Charnley (1911-1982) is considered to be the Father of Total Hip Replacement. In the early 1960s, Sir Charnley used a metal stem for the hip bone and polyethylene cup for the joint cavity.

I remember being a member of the surgical team that performed what was apparently the first hip replacement in Philadelphia when I was a young intern. My job was to hold the leg up during the procedure. What I remember most is that it was a long procedure and when my arm got tired, I got permission to support the leg on my shoulder. Even though I had assisted open heart surgery before, a leg on my shoulder is the one that sticks in my mind. It was a novel procedure at that time.

Today, practically all major joints can be replaced with metal and with excellent outcomes. So the 20th-century saw Americans take the lead away from Europeans in research and innovations. Many advances in imaging techniques, laboratory tests and newer surgical techniques were also led by Americans. World class academic institutions and research centers sprung up across the United States. The focus was on diseases which previously had poor outcomes or had been incurable. Positive results began to show. Academic institutions recruited the best researchers from all over the world, further strengthening research efforts and ultimately improving the lives of thousands and thousands of people worldwide.

With newer drugs and procedures, Americans enjoyed the best health care in the globe. But it came with a high price tag. The cost of health care skyrocketed and medicine became big business.

Chapter Twenty-Five

The Business of Medicine

Medical practice was strictly a service for thousands of years and it remained a science and an art through all that time. Physicians were paid a fee directly by the patients. That started to change with the introduction of insurance companies for medical practice.

In early 1920s, some insurance companies were established to cover medical costs after accidents and soon some hospitals introduced prepaid coverages for hospital admissions. It could be said that it was and is primarily an American-made phenomena of the 20th-century. In 1929, Blue Cross insurance started in Texas to cover a patient's hospital expenses. That expense for one day in the hospital was six dollars. Now it is in the thousands of dollars. In 1948, Blue Shield began to cover doctor's fees and outpatient expenses. Many employers started to pay for health insurance premiums as a benefit to their employees. Other insurance companies sprang up with similar policies. Even then, thousands and thousands of people were not covered and could not afford hospital expenses, especially those who were unemployed or retired. In 1965, the United States government created Medicare to cover those who are over sixty-five and Medicaid for the indigent and poor.

With a combination of private insurance, Medicare and Medicaid, the majority of the population was covered. This resulted in a sea of changes in medical practice. With the availability of coverage for expenses, more people started seeking medical help, causing a greater need for doctors, nurses, and hospitals. More hospitals were opened in urban and in rural areas. Most hospitals in America were funded (or partially funded) by government, universities, and nonprofit organizations and religious institutions. The system, however, was not prepared to meet the demand and the tremendous need for doctors and nurses. The American Medical Association chose to recruit doctors from abroad. In 1967, a certifying examination was set up to select qualified candidates. The Examination for Certifying Foreign Medical Graduates

(ECFMG) was conducted in different parts of the world. Those who passed the examination could come to the United States for a five-year period of internship and residency. This was a way to supply doctors to large hospitals. Nurses were also allowed to come in a similar fashion. Most of these professionals came from countries, including India, China, Philippines and South Korea. Still, it was thought to be a temporary solution, but in reality, if graduates from foreign countries were sent back, the doctor shortage would only grow worse. The solution was to allow them to become immigrants.

Along with expansion of hospitals and medical coverage, the cost of healthcare soared. Drug companies charged heavy prices for the new drugs. While major pharmaceutical companies originated in countries, particularly in Canada, the U.K and all of Europe, they branched out and hiked-up the cost of drugs sold in America. To bring down the costs, the government introduced two changes to medical reimbursement plans in the mid 1980s. Until then, hospitals were paid on a per-diem basis whether the length of stay was justified or not. Under the new rule, the payment was changed to a system called DRG (Diagnosis Related Group). Basically, there was a set pay for each diagnosis, whether patients stayed one week or four weeks. DRG had some temporary success. Then hospital administrators found a way to circumvent the new rules.

Another change was the way doctors were reimbursed. Instead of paying for whatever was billed, a new system called RVUs (Relative value Units) was established where a level was assigned based on time spent, complexity of the problem and how detailed the documentation was. The concept was good, but again, there was a way to make a four-page report a level-5 examination using drop down menus and "cut and paste." Yet such measures failed to bring down costs. Uninsured numbers stayed high as did drug costs. Until then, hospitals were mostly non-profit oriented. Suddenly, for-profit entities came into the market. Competition ensued and hospitals started building five-star style buildings with heavy marketing further escalating the cost of care. The ultimate result was, the richest country in the world had the highest percentage of uninsured among developed counties.

As business interest started taking over the practice of medicine, the attitude of hospital administrators started to change. They wanted to support specialties which would bring more money at the expense of those not so glamorous but essential—for example, primary care. They preferred to invest more in procedure-oriented departments because that generated more income. For insurance companies, it became the provider that had an encounter with their clients.

By the end of 20th-century, cries to change the system became louder and louder. Patients, more than anyone else, agreed that something should be done to improve health care delivery and manage price control. Many were not eligible to buy insurance coverage if they had a pre-existing disease, such as cancer, diabetes and heart diseases. Insurance companies were "cherry picking and lemon dropping" because of a profit motive. By the end of the century, thirty-seven million Americans did not have coverage.

To me, it was an unpardonable situation for the most prosperous nation on earth. So far, in the 21st-century the issue remains the same.

2001-2100, A.D.

TWENTY-FIRST CENTURY
Computerized Technology Dominates

Chapter Twenty-six

From Bedside to Desktop

The 21st-century began with domination of computer technology over all walks of life and medicine was no exception. In the first decade itself, the U.S. Federal Government mandated that all hospitals and major clinics change medical documentation from paper to electronic medical records. This included all doctor and nurse reports as well as ordering drugs, tests, laboratory, and other reports. There were some good, bad, and ugly outcomes.

During clinic visits or bedside visits, a doctor was forced to type notes during the encounter. The criteria for billing was based on how detailed the notes were. To achieve this, the doctor needed to type while talking. The unintended outcome is that a doctor is looking at the computer screen rather than making eye contact with the patient. Since orders are written on the computer, drug duplications can be avoided. Warnings on drug interactions or serious side effects can be displayed on the screen. The notes can be sent to other doctors, clinics or even other hospitals immediately. Another advantage is legibility of notes. Doctors are notorious for bad handwriting! These are all good changes.

The new system changed the way ward rounds are conducted. Predicated on my experience while practicing and teaching medicine in America, this is the workable system I knew: rounds started at the nurse's station where the doctor got the nurse's report. This gave vitals signs, intake/output, how the patient slept or other changes that happened during the previous night. This activity was not merely information gathering, it was team building. Now all the information is in the computer, and the doctor can retrieve it even before arriving at the hospital. The bad part is, the doctor/nurse interaction and team spirit are lost.

Now, this is probably the ugly part. During the office visit, hardly any eye contact with the patient occurs because the doctor is looking at a computer screen during that time. There may or may not be a cursory hands-on examination. These days, how often we hear patients complain that the doctor never looked at them. In my practice, I saw a lot of chronic back-pain patients who had been to several doctors before. Time and again I heard the patient say, "You are the first doctor to touch my back!" So, what happened to the age-old custom of empathetic look, listen and touch, the cardinal steps of art of medicine? Is this an ugly outcome of digitalization?

The pharmacological revolution emerged in the latter half of the 20th-century and continued in the current century. The quest among Pharma companies and universities was to improve efficacy and reduce side effects of existing drugs. They also started looking for new drugs to treat diseases like cancer, diabetes, heart diseases and many others. Investigations proceeded to find a cure for diseases that were considered incurable, such as multiple sclerosis, Alzheimer's, A.L.S. Genetic mapping to identify defective genes causing congenital diseases led to genetic engineering techniques to remove defective genes. A new set of biological and bio-similar drugs for difficult-to-treat diseases, such as rheumatoid arthritis, lupus, and Crohn's disease proved effective.

The pharmacological approach changed from "one size fits all" to individualized treatment. Medicine learned that a particular medicine good for one person may not be good for another. There is different effectiveness based on sex and race and family history. Overall, genetic profiling to select the right medicine became part of personalized medicine.

Then newer surgical techniques, such as surgery through a small incision developed to replace several open surgeries, including open heart and abdominal surgeries. Surgery to correct congenital abnormalities in the newborn and sometimes when the baby is in the womb were introduced. Newer tests and procedures were available to improve diagnostic accuracy.

Perhaps there are two areas which require attention of both the public and government. One is the number of uninsured or under-insured in the country. According to National Center for Health Statistics, forty-eight million (16%) in the U.S population were in this category in 2010. A significant portion of uncompensated care came from this group. This adds to the cost for healthcare. After the Affordable Care Act of 2010 was enacted, the number of uninsured reduced to twenty-nine million (9%) by 2018. Another area needing attention is public health. Are we spending and paying more attention to individual solutions for diseases and ignoring public health? Had we focused on public health, we would have been better prepared for a pandemic like Covid-19 that struck and rapidly spread early in the year 2020.

As the medical practice moved from bedside to desktop, there were some changes in attitude. To treat a disease, science alone may be sufficient; but to treat a patient it takes science and art. If doctors focus on treating a disease and not the patient, the art of medicine becomes irrelevant. Another trend is the rush to prolong life at any cost without regard to quality of life if the patient survives. Respecting and encouraging a Living Will to dictate what each person desires to be done if irreversible changes impact the survivor's quality of life is advisable.

Is dramatic change in how medicine is practiced in the future now on the horizon? Will medicine become a science leaving art out of it? Will "citizen doctor" consult I.B.M 's Dr. Watson for diagnosis and Dr. Google for the treatment? Only time will tell.

2020, A.D.

THE FUTURE OF MEDICINE
As I See It

Chapter Twenty-Seven

The Future of Medicine — As I See It

One hundred years ago, no one may have imagined that before the end of the century, man would walk in space or walk on the surface of the moon. Similarly, can we imagine that one day we will be able to prevent the aging process? Can nano robots get into the cells and prevent degenerative changes in the brain, internal organs, or joints? Can genetic engineering prevent the aging process? Will it help humans to live for hundreds of years or even for eternity? Is it a science fiction? Is Mother Earth ready for it?

The search for new drugs to improve present ones or to cure diseases that cannot currently be cured is in full swing. With grants to universities from National Institute of Health, philanthropists and Pharma industry, we are making tremendous progress. So, search for the cause of cancer and cure for cancer is within the realm of reality. Drugs may be prescribed based on genetic profile. Bioengineering research may lead to movement of paralyzed muscles. Genetic mapping may be able to predict diseases a person may encounter. Genetic engineering may then be able to correct defective genes which cause congenital abnormalities. Advanced research may be able to destroy disease-causing cells selectively. The good old magic bullet theory envisioned one-hundred years ago may not be a pipe dream after all.

The Covid-19 epidemic of the 21st-century forced clinics to resort to telemedicine. Many, especially seniors, did not accept it because it lacks in-person contact. However, millennials may accept it more willingly because of their familiarity with digital communication. So in the future, many outpatient visits may be virtual, especially in rural areas. Mobile health trucks can function as outpatient clinics equipped to perform basic tests like X-Rays, EKG, simple blood and urine tests. With the help of a nurse, a physician sitting in a remote hospital can listen to heart and lung sounds, check the affected areas and come to a diagnosis and prescribe treatment.

The biggest change expected in the near future is introduction of Artificial Intelligence. This is intended to mimic human intelligence faster and more efficiently and is expected to exceed human capability. The result is a data-driven approach with algorithms and charts. A patient's X-Rays and scans can be compared with thousands of other images and be given an opinion. AI can instantly review hundreds of reference articles and give a summary of opinions. These reports can warn about subtle as well as complex associations in a patient's case, all with a click of a button. The report can suggest safer and more effective treatment options.

There is another side to this progression, a human side which starts at bedside. Medicine is not an exact science. So many variables and biases go into making a diagnosis and selecting treatment. A human connection established between two individuals, doctor and patient, is the starting point. A computer or an algorithm cannot come as a third player. It may be acceptable as an assisted tool. During Tinsley Harrison's lifetime (1900-1978), the renowned professor at the University of Alabama's Medical College updated and edited five editions of his textbook, Principles of Medicine. Still well-known and cited today, Principles of Medicine is now in its twentieth edition. In the preface to an early edition, Harrison said that in treating the suffering, he (the physician) needs technical skills, scientific knowledge and human understanding. Specifically, he said, "The physician also uses these with courage, with humility and with wisdom."

Posthumously, Dr. William Osler, a respected physician and one of the founders of Baltimore's Johns Hopkins Hospital, continues to be quoted in medical journals even now, one-hundred years beyond his death. Educators often advise students of Osler's legacy as I did during the span of my fifty-year career as a practitioner and teacher. Osler emphasized that medicine is taught and learned at the beside, more than in the classroom. With a dozen or more texts written by or about Osler, a favorite available today is The Quotable Osler who was known to say, "Listen to your patient. He is telling you the diagnosis. Listen not only to symptoms; also, their fears."

Through all the changes and breakthroughs of the past and the future of medicine, a basic characteristic remains: Human connection is essential to treat the disease. That is the joy of clinical medicine. Computers or Artificial Intelligence cannot take that away.

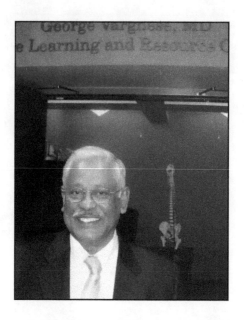

A youthful dream of becoming a doctor
in America carried George Varghese from
a village in India to the U.S. and national
prominence as a medical specialist, diagnostician, educator and visionary. Dr. Varghese
was honored with the Lifetime Achievement
Award from the American Academy of Physical Medicine and Rehabilitation. He is Professor Emeritus at University of Kansas Medical
Center. He lives with his wife Molly in Kansas
City where they raised three children.